T0353692

RETURNING TO PERFECT

Created to Heal...

SUSAN FARAH

BALBOA.PRESS
A DIVISION OF HAY HOUSE

Balboa Press books may be ordered through booksellers or by contacting:

Balboa Press
A Division of Hay House
1663 Liberty Drive
Bloomington, IN 47403
www.balboapress.com
844-682-1282

Because of the dynamic nature of the Internet, any web addresses or links contained in this book may have changed since publication and may no longer be valid. The views expressed in this work are solely those of the author and do not necessarily reflect the views of the publisher, and the publisher hereby disclaims any responsibility for them.

The author of this book does not dispense medical advice or prescribe the use of any technique as a form of treatment for physical, emotional, or medical problems without the advice of a physician, either directly or indirectly. The intent of the author is only to offer information of a general nature to help you in your quest for emotional and spiritual well-being. In the event you use any of the information in this book for yourself, which is your constitutional right, the author and the publisher assume no responsibility for your actions.

Any people depicted in stock imagery provided by Getty Images are models, and such images are being used for illustrative purposes only. Certain stock imagery © Getty Images.

Print information available on the last page.

Scripture quotations are taken from the Holy Bible, NEW INTERNATIONAL VERSION®, NIV® Copyright © 1973, 1978, 1984, 2011 by Biblica, Inc.® Used by permission. All rights reserved worldwide.

ISBN: 979-8-7652-5877-4 (sc)
ISBN: 979-8-7652-5876-7 (e)

Library of Congress Control Number: 2024926851

Balboa Press rev. date: 02/07/2025

This book is dedicated to my husband Tom – who without, I never would have experienced this journey...

Love,
Susan

CONTENTS

CONTENTS

PROLOGUE

Life is an incredible journey full of starry nights and rainy days, rooftops and valleys, lush banquets and arid deserts.

But the most incredible journey is not one that we experience - it is one that we possess.

It is the only true possession we have - and it is amazing and awe-inspiring. That possession - "our possession" is - us. It is our body, soul and spirit, the essence of all we were created to be.

You notice I stated that *our possession is us, "we" - the essence of all we were created to be.* And not, the essence of all we *are* now.

Why?

Simple, we are not all we were created to be, at least not all the time. You see, we were created to be so much more – more than we are now and more than what we know or believe we are.

In our natural state, our full capacity we are more intricate and complex than the tiniest computer, more resilient and tough than an armored tank *and* more fragile and easily broken than spun glass.

We are a study in contradictions...

And it is in these contradictions that the truth of us is revealed. The greatest scholars could spend their entire lifetime trying to figure us out, and never finish trying.

We are unique, we are *too* unique.

There is, never was and never will be any other creature like us. We were created for a unique purpose - not just some swamp slime adapting over time into a higher form of swamp slime. But wonderfully made and intentionally designed to be all these walking, talking contradictions that can be only one thing – a reflection of the one who created us. Resilient and ever-changing beings created with limitless capabilities and endless possibilities.

Our true identity and our true purpose are revealed to each of us over time. Some understand it quickly and walk boldly sharing themselves with others every day of their life while others take a different path and don't truly discover themselves until much, much later.

Neither is wrong but, one seems so much more rewarding, doesn't it?

So fellow humans, we are not just built for survival but, we also were "created to heal."

And we have been specially prepared for both.

Does that frighten you?

Does it shock you?

Then, "Close your eyes, open your mind *and* hang on tight for the ride of your life!"

CHAPTER ONE

BUILT FOR SURVIVAL...

You've probably heard this phrase many times before, "Survival of the fittest" but did you know that it doesn't matter how fit you are?

All humans were built for survival.

From the top of our heads to the tip of our toes every minute of every day our built-in radar detector is on search to sniff out anything that is trying to destroy us.

If I was allowed only two words to describe this human phenomenon, the first would have to be - *survivor.*

And why not, since we were fashioned in the image of our creator. Why shouldn't we have his characteristics? And why wouldn't we have been designed to last a long time in perfect health with perfect well-being since it was always intended that we *would* spend an eternity conversing with this great Creator of ours.

The second word would be – *healer.*

Because to truly be able to survive anything that comes along there would have to be a mechanism in place to protect and recreate ourselves, to heal ourselves. And since we were created to protect and recreate ourselves, "Why is it so far-fetched to think that we have that same ability to affect others - to protect and heal others?"

Listen, we have sent men to the moon, perfected an artificial heart, we have invented cars without a driver and a computer that thinks for itself.

Need I say more?

And to think we did all of this with just a portion of our brain. Just think what could we do if we used all of it?

And by the way, what did you think the rest of your brain was there for?

Nothing? Or maybe just for the heck of it?

I don't think so. We are too efficiently built to have a big lump of something just lying around with nothing to do. To quote a famous movie, "It would be an awful waste of space."

So, let's look at some really interesting stuff about you, about "us". Let's take a look at what we *were* created to be.

As I mentioned before we were made in the image of our Creator for the sole purpose of fellowship, conversing and sharing - for spending time with him. To be able to do that we would need to be like him so we could communicate with him and have that communicating be satisfying on both ends. *Genesis 1:26-27.*

Sound logical?

So, man, (a human being) was created. Let's call him Adam.

Now our Creator is busy and can't spend 100% of his time with Adam so he creates a companion for Adam, let's call her Eve. Eve is also made in the image of the Creator, (let's call him God). And since we have these two beings created by God perfectly for the sole purpose of satisfying fellowship it stands to reason that their surroundings, their world, (let's call it a garden) must be perfect, too.

There are no storms, tornadoes, floods, freezing temperatures, torrid heat or humidity to worry about or distress them. The air is clean, the water is pure and the plants and trees are free from disease. There is nothing to interfere with these two beings created in the image of their Creator to last forever communing with God in a perfectly, climate-controlled healthy world. And, of course in bodies that have been specifically created to last forever, happily in fellowship with their Creator.

Sounds like Utopia, doesn't it? What happened?

Well, now here's where it starts to get tricky.

They blew it!

Tens of thousands of people for thousands of years have argued about what happened - and in the end, it doesn't matter. The why is not important only "the what" is.

And that "what" is - *suddenly the story of two perfect beings living in a perfect world no longer existed.*

Sadly, and unfortunately for us it was replaced with perfect beings built for perfect survival living in an *imperfect world – a world they were not created for.*

And we all know what happens when a boxer doesn't train, a musician doesn't practice and someone isn't prepared for what is about to happen to them – *splat!*

Roadkill…

Jump ahead several thousand years and here we are trying to figure out what happened and what to do about it. I say we are looking in the wrong direction - instead of looking for a solution, we need to understand we *are* the solution.

To comprehend this, we have to *know* who we are and what our inheritance is, what our birthright is. Understand who our father is, what our gene pool is and where we come from.

Once we understand those things then we will have the knowledge we need, when combined with our faith and multiplied by our trust; to live as heirs of the Most High - to heal ourselves and heal others.

Why do I believe this? How do I know this to be true?

Because there is no other explanation for the truth – it's just the truth. So, let's examine the truth.

In this chapter we will explore the five main "life-saving" components common to every human being on this planet no matter where or how they live, what their race, nationality or ethnic group, their religious belief or economic status. This exploration may or may not surprise you but it will definitely challenge you and I hope it will get you thinking about things you never have thought about before.

One disclaimer before we get started.

Medically speaking, this could get a little complicated, but this revelation of information is not intended to be complicated. So, to diffuse the complication, I have taken the liberty of "breaking down" the cumbersome medical terms into more common language we all can understand.

I hope it suits you, here we go:

We were built for survival - we *did not* evolve to survive.

But what we did do and what we have as part of our building blocks of survival is the ability to adapt - "adaptability".

What's the difference between the two?

Well, evolve means to progress, to advance. A good example would be computers and mobile phones. Back in the 70's and 80's when we were just beginning with the "Technology Age" computers were the size of rooms and a mobile phone was a telephone in a large carrying case that was made mobile.

Look where we are now – cell phones that can be your butler and computers that can fit on the head of a pen or maybe pin. That's evolution – evolution of technology.

Adapt, (adaptability) means to adjust *and* have flexibility.

A perfect example of this is a person who is born blind or with four fingers on each hand instead of five. The person born without sight soon adapts and learns to heighten their other senses - hearing and awareness to their environment surrounding them so they can live as well as the "seeing" people around them. The same principle goes for the person born only with four fingers. Their flexibility and adaptability will allow them to learn to perform the *same tasks as someone with five fingers.*

This adaptability is a survival characteristic. It's also a human characteristic because innate objects can't adapt themselves – *a human has to develop or change the object for it to evolve.*

Hence, humans are adaptable. We haven't changed, we have adapted. We are as we were created - we have just made necessary modifications to continue to survive in the world we live in *now*.

So, let's dive right into our first discovery which is called the "Flight or Fight Response".

You may know a few things about it, but let's study it from top to bottom, back to front and beginning to end. All living creatures have some type of "fight or flight" instinctual response built into their being; the "fear" response.

Everything was created to survive - to fulfill its purpose. Whether that purpose was to conquer and tame or to be one of the links in a long food chain - all creatures have had this survival button since they were created. And when activated, this "survival mechanism" saves lives; ours and others.

Now some of these instinctual responses are quite complicated and they vary from creature to creature and from plant to plant, but what we are interested in today is what happens to you and me, to us - humans.

So, here are the basic mechanics for this survival mechanism in us. We have an area inside our brain called the hypothalamus and when stimulated from a real or perceived threat automatically sets off a series of events that prepares us for attack or retreat – "fight or flight." This response is a "wisdom" embedded in our DNA that happens without our help whether we want it to happen or not.

This flight or fight, when activated, bypasses our rational mind (where we tend to think out situations before we act and react), and moves directly into "GO". Instantaneously a number of things happen - sequences of nerve cell firings occur and chemicals such as adrenaline, nor-adrenaline and cortisol are released into our bloodstream and produce dramatic changes.

> *Our breathing gets faster, our heart rate increases and our blood pressure rises making us feel a sense of "being charged". Blood and glucose is redirected from parts*

of our body which are less important at that time (digestive and immune systems). This sudden rush of extra blood to our brain, arms, legs and muscles readies us and gives us a feeling of alertness and increased energy. It also gives us the feeling of "goose bumps" because the hairs really do stand up on end as tensed muscles pull on the skin. These tense muscles and the overall heightened energy can cause us to shake.

Oxygen increases to the lungs and our perspiration increases.

Our pupils dilate, our sight sharpens and our awareness intensifies.

We get tunnel vision, (loss of peripheral vision).

Our saliva and tear production decrease.

Auditory exclusion happens, (loss of hearing).

Our sense of pain diminishes, our fear is exaggerated and our thinking is distorted.

*We see everything through the filter of possible danger, our focus is narrowed and **fear** now becomes the lens through which we see the world.*

We are now tuned for short-term survival - not long-term consequences.

We have all heard the stories of ordinary people doing extraordinary things – a mother single-handedly lifting a car off her child pinned underneath or an elderly woman subduing a purse snatcher or beating off an attacker. All things everyday people would not be able to do under normal circumstances. Well, all of this is due to that built-in "flight or fight" survival system.

It is a perfect system. It is meant to be a perfect system – survival by retreat or battle.

It is meant to be perfect because after the danger is eliminated and the threat is gone our body is supposed to go back to its homeostatic state, (normal and calm). Thus giving us time to rest and ready ourselves for the normality of life or the next challenge.

But what happens when the danger - that threat or fear, is not an isolated incident?

What happens when it's not a car accident or you stumbling onto a burglar but it is living with a physically abusive husband or the daily financial strain manifested in losing your job, your car or your house or maybe even your family?

What about rush hour traffic five days a week, being a single mom with no education and trying to raise several children or a soldier out on the battle lines fearing death and knowing he may have to kill at a moment's notice or be killed himself?

Then there is the fight with your boss. You can't punch him out or flee – you have to stay at your desk or on the factory floor and just "handle" it. How about someone cutting you off in traffic and causing an accident that nearly demolishes your car or maybe nearly demolishes you? It's called road rage and has been known to kill.

Whether we acknowledge it or not, in the year 2025 we are in a battle daily and the battle cry is "stress".

And as you may have heard - *stress can kill you.*

We are in a world, a global community of major stressors that trigger a full activation of our fight or flight response almost continually; causing us to become aggressive, hyper-vigilant and over-reactive which puts us in counter-balance with our perfect health. This has become counter-productive to our survival and in fact, has become *the enemy* – our enemy.

Our perfect survival mechanism, that gift from our creator – has had its "go" button jammed and it's "stop" button malfunctioning for so long it has rusted shut. As a result, our bodies are not returning to the "rest" cycle to replenish and regroup.

It's like a washing machine that is stuck on the spin cycle hopelessly going around and around until the motor burns up, and then is carted away to that junkyard in the sky where all appliances, (too expensive to repair) go to rust and turn to dust.

What happens to us is the cumulative buildup of stress hormones that are not metabolized correctly but used in our bodies improperly; making us ill over time from the precise thing that was designed to save us.

Wow!

No wonder some of us feel so bad.

So, what are the warning signs of this happening and what can be done about it?

It is no surprise that the warning signs are very logical when you think about what happens during our "fight or flight – fear/stress" response. All those levels in our body that increase, if they stay at that heightened level our/your stress would look like:

Headaches, back pain, tight neck and shoulders, chronic fatigue and racing heart which can lead to: *cardiac problems, restlessness, sleep problems, tiredness, dizziness, loss of appetite, ringing in your ears, high blood pressure and too much glucose released, (weight gain and diabetes).*

And these are just the main ones. Then there are all the levels in our body that decrease. If *they stay* at that low ebb this is what our/your prolonged stress looks like:

Indigestion, stomach pain, and susceptibility to infection, autoimmune diseases like rheumatoid arthritis, lupus, allergies and problems with sexual enjoyment and/or sexual performance.

And if that wasn't enough no matter if we are talking about the high or the low levels - *these* next symptoms can manifest themselves:

Inability to get things done, increase in smoking, eating or alcohol, compulsive gum chewing, grinding teeth, crying, overwhelming sense of pressure, bossiness and criticizing others, nervousness, anxiety, feeling powerless to change things, being easily upset, feeling that there is no meaning to life, loneliness, anger, unhappiness for no reason, trouble thinking clearly, loss of sense of humor, memory loss, constant worry, lack of creativity, thoughts of running away, inability to make decisions and even post-traumatic stress disorder (PTSD).

Whew!

Who the heck wants all of those?

What do we do?

How do we reverse the effects of the miracle plan that was meant to sustain us that now has gone awry?

What do we do about this "thing" that is now killing us?

How do we take back our lives and live with the full intent in which we were created?

Honestly, I think the first thing is we have to accept the truth that this gift was designed to protect us from real life-threatening danger - *not 2025 man-made stress.*

Next, we have to accept that we were designed to survive at all costs.

This one is a little tricky because you might want to counter it by saying, "But why is our skin so fragile and easily penetrated"? Or how about when our main arteries and veins are severed and we bleed to death?

Ah-hah!

There's a difference between inherent survival systems and us taking care of our bodies so they don't get damaged beyond repair.

Did you ever watch the movie, "Death Becomes Her"?

Let that one sink in for a minute before we tackle the "what to do" part and instead let's move on to another survival system and we'll save the conclusions for a little later.

Let's talk about our immune system and the inflammatory response. This is an amazing defense system and again another example of an incredibly designed and interwoven series of events taking place in our body simultaneously.

Did you know you have a built-in "enemy-buster?

It's called your immune system and it is constantly on the lookout for anything in your body "that it believes is, or that recognizes as" foreign and harmful - and then it automatically defends against it.

It is the Army, Navy, Air Force and Marines all rolled into one.

It's your "Special Forces" - your "Black Ops" living only to seek and destroy. And just like the troops that defend our country are broken down into different departments of the Armed Services, so is our immune system. Let's call our immune system the "Big I" for this lesson and talk about all these different departments of the "Big I" that were stamped onto your DNA from Day One.

So, here we go.

Your troops live to seek out and destroy antigens and antigens are substances, (usually proteins) on the surface of cells, viruses, fungi, or bacteria. Then there are non-living substances like toxins, chemicals, drugs and foreign particles (such as a splinter), which can also be antigens. In addition, your own body's cells have proteins too that are antigens, but your immune system learns to see these as normal and usually does not react against them.

That's a lot of antigens, (enemies) the "Big I" has to deal with, isn't it?

And because of that there are several kinds of immunity that our body has working simultaneously and together to keep us healthy. These are: innate, acquired, passive and components in your blood.

Innate (or nonspecific immunity), is the defense system we all were born with. It is part of our natural health and when working perfectly helps to keep our bodies in a constant state of well-being. It is our first line of defense and was created in the form of barriers that keep harmful materials from entering our bodies. Examples include: cough reflex, stomach acid, skin, mucus – which traps bacteria and small particles and enzymes in tears and skin oils.

Innate immunity also has a protein chemical form – innate humoral immunity. An example of this is interferon and interleukin-1, (which causes fever). If an antigen can get past "the front line" it is then attacked and destroyed by other parts of the "Big I".

I see you have already guessed what an incredible and highly sophisticated creation we are.

And, we're just getting started!

Next, we have <u>acquired</u> immunity which is immunity that develops with exposure to various antigens (foreign bodies), during our lifetime. In a nutshell: our bodies build a defense – a defensive system of stone walls, high fences and moats to block illnesses.

A good example is what happens when a healthcare professional is exposed to bacteria. Their body builds antibodies to act as an "anti-magnetic field" to stop the bacteria from making them ill. So, they don't catch everything their patients have.

Nurses and doctors totally understand this one!

Then there's <u>passive</u> immunity which is the antibodies produced in a body other than our own. Examples include babies who are born with antibodies transferred through the placenta from their mother, (these usually disappear between ages six and twelve months). And we can't forget injections of antiserums which contain antibodies formed by another person or an animal and provide immediate but not long-lasting protection. Tetanus antitoxins and immune serum globulin which is given for hepatitis exposure are other examples of passive immunity.

Lastly, let's talk about the <u>immunity contained in our blood</u>.

We have certain types of white blood cells, proteins and chemicals such as antibodies, complement proteins and interferon. Some of these directly attack foreign substances and others team-up and work together to help the immune system cells.

There are two very important types of white blood cells, (lymphocytes) and they are broken down into B and T type lymphocytes.

- B lymphocytes become cells that produce antibodies which "team-up" and make it easier for the immune cells to destroy "the enemy".
- T lymphocytes attack antigens directly and help control the immune response and release chemicals which control the entire immune system.

Pretty impressive, isn't it?

Not tadpole material – this is intentional, purposeful and well thought out by an omnipotent being.

Truly, what a magnificent creation we are!

Can you see how our immune system was assembled for our survival and when fully intact and operational was intended to keep us going for a long, long time?

But, what happens when something goes wrong? Or when something interferes with this survival immune system of ours?

Well, instead of being an efficient lifesaver it becomes excessive, lacking or inappropriate. Which is bad news for us, it stops doing its' job resulting in immune disorders such as:

Allergies (overreactions to harmless substances), anaphylaxis (life-threatening allergic reaction like bee stings or peanuts), autoimmune disorders (antibodies form against our body's own tissue and attack – Diabetes Mellitus Type I, rheumatoid arthritis and systemic lupus) and immunodeficiency disorders – the lack of the protection of our immune system leading to development of opportunistic diseases and even death which can either be inherited or acquired, (HIV/AIDS).

A really wide range - from nuisances to life-threatening, wouldn't you say? That's why our immune system is so important to us.

In addition, another important role of our immune system is to identify and eliminate tumors. There are a number of reasons why tumors grow in our body: viruses that actually cause cancer (human papillomavirus), high levels of proteins of normal cells (tyrosinase at high levels transform certain skin cells into melanomas) and mutated proteins that normally regulate our cell growth and our survival. What the immune system is designed to do is to destroy these abnormal cells using our "killer T cells" and "helper T cells".

But what happens if they get past the "Big I"?

If that happens - they go on to become cancers.

How do they do that?

Basically, *their DNA tells them they must survive*, so *their* "survival" mode kicks in and uses any means possible to avoid being destroyed. The cancers themselves grow by either their own growth system or by damaging the proteins that normally block metastasis, (the spread of) cancer cells.

Anything that decreases the immune system; poor diet, lack of sleep and rest, the normal aging process, certain medications, diseases that suppress the immune system and lack of Vitamin D can interfere with our body's defense to eliminate tumors.

A lot to think about and process, isn't it?

We also have another process going on in our bodies. It is called inflammation and is one of the *first* responses of our immune system to infection. This part of our immune system is a perfect example of an army fighting a tactical battle.

Think back to when you have fallen, hit the floor hard, gotten a bruise and a nasty cut. To the naked eye it looks like - redness, swelling, heat and pain, but to the "Big I" it is the battle cry to deploy warriors such as: white blood cells, extra body fluids, increased blood flow and a host of specialized chemicals that attack, suppress, clean-up and promote healing to the injured body part.

And remember your body does this immediately - without you having to think a thought.

In addition, we have the scouts, (phagocytes) that float around patrolling for the enemy and trapping it for destruction. Without inflammation wounds and infections would never heal, and in some cases would jeopardize our survival.

Ironically, chronic inflammation, (long-term or repeated) can lead to diseases and even cancer. Boy that "sort-term is great but long-term is terrible" situation again. And again you might ask, "What can we do"?

Keep reading...

The next process I am going to name "short and sweet" and it's called collateral circulation.

It takes less than a minute to explain, but it is a mighty gun in our arsenal of survival.

Simply put, it is when our bodies have made more than one pathway, often several, to supply blood to an organ or large area of our body.

A perfect example of this is when someone suffers a heart attack and the main artery is blocked. Luckily, the body has already built up a network of small contributories in the surrounding heart tissue to supply enough oxygenated blood to survive and heal.

You can compare this to the Mississippi River being blocked and the surrounding small rivers and streams compensate and then are able to supply just enough water to keep the fish, wildlife and plants alive.

Our bodies build this collateral circulation automatically over years. That is why quite often an older person may have a better chance of surviving a heart attack than a younger person. The older person has had time to build this system - where it is not yet available in the younger person. Again, we were built to survive.

Do you know what keeps our bodies running and our brains thinking?

Sugar...

Well actually, something called glucose the body's form of sugar. Again, this is a highly complicated chain of events, but for us we are using the microwave version. Everything we eat (consume), breaks down into glucose, (some fatty acids which the heart prefers).

Why?

Because, this is what the body uses for every system and every process; *it's the body's energy source*. Glucose is like gasoline, electricity, oil, gas, propane, windmills and solar panels all rolled into one.

We all know that the foods we eat are divided up into three classes – proteins, fats and sugars. But no matter how complex the items we are eating - they will be broken down into the simplest form; sugar (glucose), so the body can use it.

But what happens if we eat too much and there is too much for the body to use right then?

This is what is so amazing, it just doesn't disappear. Our body converts it into a substance that can be stored – fat. (Maybe to some of us this isn't so amazing but dangerous).

Now everyone has at least a little fat on them, we need to in case of an emergency. The body stores the glucose as fat so it always has "fuel" to keep every part and every action going because without glucose, (just like oxygen or water) the body will die.

What is unhealthy for us is if we overeat every day and - then every day we are storing that fat.

The "why" you already know, there is nowhere for that fat to go unless we make an effort to "rev up" the furnace and make our body need more fuel, (fat – glucose) to burn. So, it just hangs around, sticks to us and builds up into layers of "wiggly, jiggily glump" that we have to drag around with us. And since it's lazy and has nothing else to do it also decides to clog up our arteries and push our blood pressure through the roof!

Now, something that I learned in nursing school that totally mesmerized me at the time was what happens when someone is not able to eat. Whether the person is sick and can't eat, stranded somewhere without food or they are purposefully not eating - their perfect body built for survival will automatically begin a chain of chemical reactions which breaks down the stored glucose, (glycogen) in their fat tissues to make the energy necessary to maintain all the functions of their body to keep them alive.

Amazing!

This isn't the body's first choice of energy - but it works.

How long will it work? Well, as long as there is a fat reserve.

What happens after that, when the fat is gone?

In the next phase our body will break down the protein, (muscles) to squeeze out as much glucose for energy as it can get. But because it takes more protein to produce the same amount of energy, we will start to get weaker and may not function as well, (remember the heart and many other vital organs are muscle). The body will continue to do this as long as it can to keep us alive. It will use everything it can and do whatever it must do to continue to exist.

That's what I call survival!

These are the top five lifesavers we are going to talk about for now, but to be perfectly honest and totally factual - there are many more. In fact, the entire human body in itself is one huge series of surviving actions, all inter-related, co-dependent and (hopefully), all working in harmony.

If our body was a TV show it would never run out of ideas, plots or subplots. It would make "Survivor" look like kindergarten.

That is because every aspect of every part of our body down to the tiniest molecule is constantly in the state of pursuing its purpose of "survival of the creation"; maintaining perfect existence towards an eternity of co-existing with its creator, its source - God.

That's what it was created to do. That's what's stamped in its DNA, our DNA. And that is what it will do until it can't do it anymore.

Unlimited potential with unlimited possibilities...

But, why the tenacity, why the persistence?

Why did our creator go to such great lengths to create us to last forever?

And why don't we? Or do we?

If we have been built for ultimate survival and our potential is unlimited, limitless - what else is possible?

What else are we capable of having the ability to do or the ability of being that we are not now? What else is there?

And, how can we get our body back into its perfect harmony and properly working so we can tap into "the other" that we aren't yet aware of?

What can we do?

What must we understand to be all that we were meant to be?

Is there only one reason why we were created or are there more?

And, I am sure you have your own questions, too.

Why is there so much sickness?

Why do I feel bad so much of the time?

Why do children die?

And the list goes on and on...

As you ponder these questions, let's learn a little more about this perfect instrument – *us*.

CHAPTER TWO

THE HEALING BODY

Did you ever ask yourself these questions, "If we are created in God's image and God's image is perfect then why isn't everyone born perfect? Why are some people born with mental, emotional or physical defects?"

I have.

Over these 71 years of my life's journey I have seen a lot and experienced a lot more but still, it is only recently that I have come to understand we are talking about two different things; born perfect by some scale of perfection 1-100% and "born perfect - for our life purpose".

If we realize this difference, then it's easier to understand why everyone *has* to be different. Why some are born with defects or illness, why some live a very short life and some live to be very old - and even to understand why some can do hurtful and harmful things that seem to go against God's very nature.

So, let's talk about how this works. Let's begin with: "We were made in the image of God."

I know we have already established that, but what does "image of God" mean exactly? Well, one definition of image is that an image is a copy. So, if we are a copy of God, what does *that* look like?

Have you ever made a copy of something (say a letter,) on a copy machine? What was the result?

You should have two identical letters, an original and a copy with that being the only difference. Same with us, God made us to be a pure reflection of him - a mirror image that he could converse with, spend time with and build a relationship with, forever.

At this point there would be about 50 different religions, sects, theologians with their etiologies and doctrines screaming.

Well guess what?

We are going to go right past that by dismissing it all. This is not about religion - this is about truth.

The truth is - none of those things matter.

We have wasted time, money, lives and purposes letting those things get in the way. We have let those things matter more than the truth, which is: *we are spiritual beings created by God in his image - a copy of himself, the "Great I AM" – the Alpha and Omega, the beginning and* the end.

We are the "Great I AM" too, made perfectly.

It <u>cannot</u>, <u>not</u> be so.

He did this so we could be like him on earth, to <u>act</u> like him on earth and to fulfill our purpose, created to be his assistant, created to work hand in hand to create this world and the lives of the individuals who live in it. That's our job.

No one knows the true power we possess.

We were born with it.

We have the potential for it, but are just lacking the knowledge of it!

It's time we unmask the hidden mysteries of our mind and our body – the hidden mysteries of our soul, our inner light and our inner knowing and discover the gifts we possess.

It's time we reunite with our natural well-being, the well-being and perfection of God.

This parallel perfect version of you already exists. It's ready for you to live and is only limited by *your* thinking, your thoughts – *your old beliefs.*

I've read the bible many times and debated with people about Creation, but last night I read something that finally clicked with me. I am sure I've heard this in church during a message at least once, but obviously I just let it rush over me and did not absorb it as we all tend to do. This is what I read:

In the Book of Genesis is the story about Adam and Eve and the Garden (I am paraphrasing now), and it says that once they had eaten of the Tree of Knowledge and *knew* the difference between good and evil God banished them from the Garden.

It was their punishment, but it was also <u>necessary</u> because - *they could not eat from the Tree of Life and live forever like God.*

Wow!

This means when they were in the Garden and innocent there was only good (no evil), they could live forever and they could eat from the Tree of Life because they were made in God's image - perfect. They were good and *incapable of evil, incapable to do evil.*

But once they *knew* evil they were *capable* of evil.

"Ah-hah!"

Let me say that again – *"Once they knew evil they were capable of evil."*

They <u>had</u> to be thrown out of the Garden. They had to be thrown out of their "perfect world". The only world their body knew how to live in - the Garden, *not outside the Garden.*

So now they were cast into a hostile world which they knew nothing about and their "being" was not meant to live in. A world they weren't prepared for - a world their body was not prepared for.

Since then, we (their descendants in some fashion), have been on a downward spiral - physically, mentally, emotionally and spiritually fighting to survive. Fighting to survive but not knowing the rules, having no playbook or instructions to go by or knowing what we were truly capable of.

We have been on a treasure hunt for the "Fountain of Youth" without a map!

But even though all of this is true, our perfectly-built machine is still trying to survive "perfectly" in an imperfect world. No wonder we are always at odds with ourselves.

To understand all of this more fully let's talk a little bit further about us humans and discover a little bit more about this machine of ours.

We have a system in our body that without our conscious thought - beats our hearts, breathes air into our lungs and blinks our eyes. Just think what would happen if you had to tell yourself to breathe every breath or tell your heart to pump every beat - it would take all your time just to do that and...

What if you forgot? What would happen when you fell asleep?

Again, survival happens *beyond our control* because we were meant for *greater things than just to survive.*

Did you know that the only part of the human body that does not heal itself is a tooth?

Okay, how about the rest of our body parts that were created for our survival? How about our kidneys, liver and lymph nodes, which all filter impurities and poisons from our body – again, imperative to our survival.

How about our heart (circulatory system), that works one way while we are in the womb and the then second we are born and breathe air for the first time - totally reverses itself so we can survive outside in the real world.

Then there's our bone marrow which is crucial for replenishing our blood – again, without which we could not survive. Our thyroid regulates our metabolism which is necessary for the breakdown and use of glucose, medications, vitamins and minerals – any and all energy resources.

How about the amazing phenomenon of breathing in air, breathing out carbon dioxide which is exactly what trees and plants need to live and then *they* discard oxygen – the exact thing *we* need to survive.

Now that is efficiency - and utterly amazing!

What an incredibly perfect way to guarantee survival of two unrelated species. Think about the chances of that - the chance that this could randomly happen on its' own accord.

Impossible!

It was a well-crafted plan down to the tiniest detail and then implemented perfectly.

What else?

Isn't that enough? No?

How about this…

In our natural state our bodies are perfectly capable of health and well-being all the time. Get a cut, the cut is healed and new skin appears as long as nothing interferes with this natural process. Break a bone – immobilize it, (let it rest) and without outside interference it heals all by itself. *I Corinthians: 19*

Still asking why there is so much sickness and diseases? Still telling yourself this is too hard to believe?

Still denying the truth?

What is the truth?

The truth is that when humans were first created our bodies were meant to remain perfect in that setting and that time, forever. What setting and what time and what happened to change it?

Those are things that can be debated forever – again a big waste of time.

What *is* important is that it now is a different setting and time which means we are now like *a fish out of water*. Our bodies are trying to maintain health and well-being and to survive in a world and a time that they *weren't* meant to do it in. As a result, *no amount* of adapting can compensate for the vast disparities between the two.

Let's name a few of these disparities, just a few things out of hundreds maybe thousands that are different now and that interfere with this natural ability to heal ourselves and to survive.

How about clean air, clean water, no pesticides or insecticides, no freeze-drying or hydrogenated foods, no cars running on gasoline, no plastics made out of oil, no problems with the "O-Zone" layer, no microwaves, no steroids, no artificial hormones or antibiotics pumped into our food, no MSG and no GMO's.

Since there was no electricity and no radios, televisions or computers when the sun went down people went to sleep and when the sun came up they awoke and did a full days' physical labor, (whatever that meant for them).

Next comes the sleep and exercise cycles which kept their bodies in working condition and rejuvenated for the next day. No telephones, no fax machines and no critical deadlines – except natural ones such as when to plant (sow), and when to harvest (reap).

Stress (like we know it), was not a word or a reality that existed. Life was not easy but it was natural and what could be done in a day was done. And tomorrow - was left until tomorrow.

Words like life, liberty, freedom, conscience, fairness, family, community, honor and trust were not just meaningless words strewn about like so much compost. They were the substance that held everything together keeping the stress out and the worry at bay.

So, what do we do since we are now in the year 2025 and people are what they are? The world and the planet are now in the condition they are in and we have technology: "two for bad, one for good".

Now what?

As Dorothy is told in "The Wizard of Oz" by the Mayor of Munchkinland, she must start at the beginning. So, we too, will take the munchkins advice and start with "us" and the *beginning.*

Our body has an innate sense of knowing how to heal itself. Unimpeded it is capable of healing and maintaining itself in a homeostatic level until its use is over. Our job is to remove the obstacles from its path and stay out of its way because *"we are our own worst enemy".*

It is not illness and disease that is the culprit.

It is not catastrophic circumstances or even genetic or hereditary genes that destroy our ability to live in a natural state of health and well-being. It is us. "Us" as a collective body and "us" - each and every one individually.

We are the villains.

We have taken on the illness and the sickness of the world and made it a part of who we believe we are. *We* all wear the mark of hypochondria in some fashion.

How can we help it?

Watch the television, read the magazines and turn on your computer and really see all the things our minds are bombarded with every waking moment.

"Do you feel blue? You're depressed – take a pill".

"Can't sleep? You have insomnia – take a pill".

"Tired?

Drink this 5-hour concoction of chemicals - it will fix you right up".

"Don't have this car, look like this air-brushed model or live in this *up-to-your-neck-in-debt* house?"

"LOSER..."

"You might as well give up – take a pill, get drunk or go eat a 3,000 calorie, triple-decker, fat-oozing, giant full-meal deal."

Quit being a victim of advertising!

Quit letting others tell you who you are, what you are and what's best for you. Quit believing everything you read on the internet and on Facebook. You do know a large part of it is false - not true, a fabrication and a lie, right?

And throw away the labels.

Not the ones on your boxes and jars of food – *the ones you are allowing others to label you with!*

Stop being a walking corpse!

Did you ever wonder why when you drink a sweet, soft drink or eat a donut or a handful of potato chips and it doesn't satisfy you – you want more, much more? So, you end up eating thousands of empty calories and feel sluggish or "fat" a short while later?

Why?

It wasn't what your body needed, so your body has not been satisfied. Your body will continue to signal you that it's not satisfied until *it is* satisfied - not until *you* are satisfied.

Did you hear that? Did you understand what I just said?

Your body will continue to signal you until it is satisfied - not until YOU are satisfied.

And guess what?

We are not just talking about food here. Our bodies are always trying to bring itself back to our natural state of health and well-being. We're talking about your body, too - remember?

I said *our* (your), natural state not our sister's or brothers' natural state, not the beauty queen's down the street, not like some multi-million, dollar athlete or paper-thin model in Vogue.

Trying to be like them, trying to be like someone else - *is not being you.* And has nothing to do with you!

Doing what they do, eating what they eat, pumping up or throwing up like they do - is not being you in your natural state of health and well-being for the purpose inherent to *you.* So, all you are doing by imitating them is satisfying no one and making some advertiser richer.

It has nothing to do with *satisfying you — bringing YOU back to YOUR perfect.*

Hello, is anybody home?

Stop looking at others and start looking inward and upward and let your body, mind, soul and spirit connect. This way the playing field is leveled. *You are on even ground the place you must be in to return back to your perfect.*

Hmm, when you feel tired what do you do? Drink some caffeine – a coffee or a Mountain Dew?

Do you pop a pill or slap yourself in the face a few times and push yourself to keep going and going and going until a cold or the flu hits you? Do you force yourself to stay up and watch a movie, google or tweet something on the computer late into the night? Do you work all day and then work all night, too?

If so, what happens the next day – a fight with your spouse or boss? Or maybe it's a rotten day at the office with people snapping at you and you snapping back at them. Or worse yet, a fender-bender, a fall, a slip of the knife as you were cutting vegetables and now you have to deal with the insurance companies, stitches, pain and bills you can't pay.

And for what?

It all could have been avoided. Your body was telling you to *sleep* and you ignored your inner physician and - poof!

You sabotaged yourself and now you are in a jam – a big one.

As I was writing this last paragraph I was reminded of my dad. Now he lived to be almost 80 years old and was rarely sick until the last year of his life. He had only been in the hospital once at age 45 for a hernia operation, (trying to pick up something he shouldn't) and in the ER once when he sliced his finger on the tractor blade, (again doing something he shouldn't have been doing).

But what I remember most about him was whenever he felt a cold coming on or some flu symptoms he would sleep. In fact, he didn't just want to sleep - he also didn't want to eat or be bothered at all. Just let him sleep - and we did.

He knew what he needed – he was listening to his inner signal. He was allowing his body to do what it was naturally supposed to do which was getting back into alignment through rest and sleep - the body's rejuvenator.

He listened, he paid attention.

Our bodies were (and should be now), programmed to have all the energy and vitality needed to accomplish what it is supposed to accomplish for that *one* day. This is how we were created, and this is how we have been designed.

The plan was that we would accomplish our day's activities, (what was needed for *that* day) go to sleep, get the proper amount of rest so our energy bucket would be full again and *then* have all the energy and vitality needed to think, move, work, create and love for the *next* day.

Each day the cycle is complete in itself - *perfect*.

Remember, we are biological - not "robot"ical.

Since we are busy-busy people now and using up all our energy for "doing"- where's the energy coming from for "healing" and rejuvenating? That's where enough rest and sleep and even extra sleep is needed otherwise you haven't given your body what it needs to do its job.

Your bucket is empty!

Again, you (we), are putting obstacles and stone walls in the body's path. We must listen to our bodies - you must listen to your body.

Our bodies have been programmed to know what we need. If we drink when we are thirsty, eat when we are hungry, sleep when we are tired, take time to rest and play and laugh and love our bodies know how to take care of us.

But they can't do it if we don't take care of them - if we don't pay attention and give them what they need. We have to stop throwing up roadblocks and putting sink holes in their path.

Now, here's another story about my dad.

He loved his sweets and was a real "meat and potatoes" type of guy. So, for this sixtieth birthday his sister baked him a double-chocolate, three-layer birthday cake and then for the main course cooked him a 2-inch thick, one-pound T-bone steak. He ate the entire steak and then, over the next two days devoured the whole cake – *himself.*

Well, what do you think happened?

Yup, the day after he finished the cake he woke up hollering in pain. The toes on his right foot hurting him so badly even the sheet touching them was unbearable.

Yes, *he* had brought gout onto himself.

You notice I didn't say he got gout or he was stricken with gout or gout sought him out and attacked him. I said he *"brought it unto himself"* - by himself. No one's body needs a pound beef steak and a three-layer chocolate cake. So, his body fought back.

Yes, I said it, *"His body fought him."*

He might as well of gotten a gun and shot himself in the foot (in a manner of speaking), it amounted to the same thing. Obstacles, interference and just plain stubbornness on his part, he wanted it so he did it - despite the consequences.

Like we all do.

We want something so we do it or get it whether it is good for us or not and *then* we try to justify it, "Oh, it's only one time" or, "It's only a little bit" or, "I deserve a treat now and again".

Well then don't get mad if you are sick now and again - you can't *reap* health if you don't *plant* health.

What did I just say? It sounded pretty good.

You can't reap health if you don't plant health.

So, if you sow sickness – guess what you are going reap?

You got it – sickness! And what about all the things we don't do - even though we know it is important and good for us?

How about those things?

We justify that, too, "I'm too tired" (oh, so *now* you are tired, huh?), or "I'll start tomorrow" or we blame someone else, "Why did you buy those cookies?" or, "Why didn't you wake me up in time?"

Blame-shifter!

What's the matter - you too good or too lazy to set the alarm or too wimpy to say no to a cookie?

Yeah, that cookie is *"really"* mean. Think about it.

And don't even say, "The devil made me do it". "P-l-e-a-s-e" - give me a break.

And let me put in a good word for pain.

Pain gets a bad rap.

Pain is not the problem - *what is causing the pain is the problem.* The pain is there to get your *attention* so you will *do something* and find out what is wrong and make the *necessary changes* so the *problem and the pain will go away.*

So, start paying attention!

We've talked quite a bit about our perfect physical health – you know the "on a scale from 1-100 how healthy we are compared to everyone else" scale. This is the concept that says everyone is supposed to be 100% healthy all the time.

Why? Because we were so perfectly made?

Well, that is a true statement. But what also is true is that we were perfectly made for the perfect world, (which doesn't exist anymore) *and* for our purpose in life. We were made for *our ultimate purpose for being on this planet at this specific time and in this specific place.*

This is where I believe the whole thing gets a bit confusing and where we get off our square.

Unless we are truly in sync with understanding our natural health and the well-being process and our purpose *and* the fact that we no longer live in a perfect world and allow all of this to work together for our good - *we are lost.*

Most of us just tend to bounce back and forth between "kinda" understanding it and having absolutely no clue. So, we think it's all a lie and that it doesn't work - that it's just some mumbo-jumbo, just something believed by the "flaky people".

So, it's time to find out how ready you truly are because this is where the believers and the risk-takers stay on the bus - and the doubters and scoffers need to get off.

Which are you?

Okay for all the passengers who stayed, here goes:

We are what we believe.

We become what we believe in.

Our life becomes what we focus on.

Anyway you slice it, it takes commitment.

So now *I* am asking you to make a commitment to ride this journey with me with an open mind and consider all the possibilities. Because if we believe in unlimited potential and the "anything pursued is possible" concept, then we can get past the "but's" and onto the miracles.

Are you ready?

Let's get going...

CHAPTER THREE

THE HEALING MIND

You have probably by now caught on to the idea that there are two parallels going on at the same time in each one of us.

Call it tangible and intangible or physical and "non-physical" – you can call it anything you want. They both exist and on a daily basis you experience both of them working in your life and if you pay attention, you can see them working in the lives of others, too.

They are not a coincidence - and they are not luck or an accident. *They are who we are and exactly as we were created.*

Again, since we still do not fully understand how they work together - it can make for confusion, emptiness and skepticism. Today hopefully we are going to come a little bit closer to a breakthrough.

The rule is there are no rules, anything is possible - and nothing is certain.

Scared?

Does that make you uncomfortable?

Good, then you are alive - and you are human.

It is our nature to try to put everything in a little box that we can label and control. Or at least that is what we think and tell ourselves we are doing.

In reality, the only thing we can control is the reality that we can't control anything and if we realize this - *then* the possibilities open up for us.

What possibilities?

Well, first the possibility that since you can't control anything it must mean nothing can control you either.

Did you hear what I just said? *Nothing can control you.*

If nothing can control you, then the realization that your potential is limitless and your possibilities are endless can manifest itself in your life. And once *this truth* is what you fully believe: *you can live a life not bound by anything*. And this knowledge has just *freed you* to be the illimitable, timeless *and* eternal person you were created to be.

That – is the power of the mind, my friend.

In previous chapters we have talked about our body in general and how it was designed to survive and heal, fashioned after our Creator. Part of this design is having mechanisms in place to heal injuries, replenish worn-out parts and circumvent our body's tendency to fight itself.

These are the tangibles, the evident, the perceivable and what we, collectively up to this point, have been willing to accept as truth.

The mind was designed, created in the same way, wonderfully created for survival - no matter what the situation or the cost.

But to understand the total picture we must first separate the "brain" from the "mind" because they are two completely different parts of who we are. We tend to lump them together which leads to many misconceptions.

Let's begin by looking first at the brain and then we will explore it's larger global self, (the mind) – the big picture.

We already know cells regenerate, dead skin falls off and new skin replaces it. A bone is broken – it mends. Stomach ulcers bleed and destroy tissue but they repair anew and are perfectly functional again.

Try to think of yourself as a super highway under construction - well actually, more like under *reconstruction*. Something is always being repaired, resurfaced and renewed and the instructions for this to happen have already been imprinted on your DNA to do this job perfectly.

Those embedded architectural plans, those flawless directions are your construction workers with their machinery and their "yield - slow down, roadwork ahead" signs all working to keep the traffic called "*your life*" moving along *without* incident.

When I studied the brain in nursing school and how it worked - I was totally fascinated!

I couldn't get enough information and devoured anything I could find to read. Imagine something so small that it can fit in the palm of your hand has the power to recall everything you have just read verbatim - which will get you that 100% on your final exam. But at the same time has the power to make you forget everything you know or think you know - which will allow you to flunk out of school.

That's our biological computer as it is sometimes called – our brain. And except for starfish, sponges, adult sea squirts and jellyfish – all creatures have a brain.

The human brain is estimated to have 15-33 billion neurons which are the key players in communicating and carrying signal pulses throughout the body causing coordinated responses to changes in the environment and the sophisticated purposeful control of our behavior.

There are names for all the chemicals, neurotransmitters and fancy molecules and cells residing in our brain, but it amounts to gobbily-gook because all we need to know is that without our brain we could not survive. And if damage happens to our brain, depending on the location - it will determine the short or long-lasting disability we could have.

That explains the differences in individuals who suffer a cerebral vascular accident, CVA or "stroke". It can manifest - as almost no damage at all *or* the total incapacity to walk, talk and communicate in any way.

Just about anything you can think of that us, (humans) do or think is controlled by, communicated through or contributed to our brain in one way or another. Any function, action, reaction or idea *and* the way we carry each of them out – our brain is responsible for. Without our brains we can't do anything because healing and survival is its' ultimate goal.

Another important thing to know about our brain is that it does not simply grow but instead it develops and matures in an intricately orchestrated sequence of stages. At each stage the mapping becomes more complex and perfected, culminating in full development.

The example of this is the difference of how a two-year old, a 10 year-old and a 21 year-old would handle a situation or process information. And since maturation is progressive, any disruption along the way of development and maturity will have consequences in physical, mental or emotional thinking and behaviors.

Interesting enough, a baby's brain has more neurons than the adult brain. Most neurons are created before birth except in two areas – the sense of smell and the capacity to store newly acquired memories.

Good thing I'd say – *babies need more neurons, they have a lot to learn.*

So, when you think of your brain, relate it to your personal computer and what your computer does when you "google" a word. Because that's pretty much what happens when you remember, ("google") how to play your favorite song on the piano, ride a bicycle or when you smell a flower and then recognize the smell is the smell of a rose - and so is its' name.

But where our brain *differs* from a computer is something called "information processing."

We just don't store information, we are capable of processing it, comparing it to past scenario's and coupled with our current needs can make a well-thought-out decision best suited to maximize our welfare – *our survival.*

This is critical for us otherwise we could have two or more parts of our body acting at cross-purposes with each other.

What if your left foot wanted to go north and your right foot wanted to go south – you could do a split and find yourself lying face-down on the sidewalk. Maybe this is slightly overly simplified, but it does explain it perfectly.

Let's go back to the "information processing" idea for a minute and test this theory. This is where it starts to get really interesting.

Let's say there are two young men – John and Joe, both born healthy and now each are eighteen years old. John grew up in a small, Midwestern town, in a middle-class home with his parents and older sister. John was an honor student, and he knew everyone in town - his life was simple and unproblematic.

Joe on the other hand grew up in the inner-city, lived in a poor tenement apartment with his mom and three younger brothers, dropped out of high school to get a job and also knew everyone in his neighborhood – especially the ones who tried to force him every day to join their gang. Life was anything but simple and unproblematic for Joe.

But what they did have in common was each knew how to flourish in their own way in their own environment. They had learned, adapted and matured their thinking to match their surroundings and their circumstances to ensure their survival.

Now, what would happen if you switched them? One day John was dropped-kicked into Joe's world and Joe was air-lifted into John's?

Could they survive – would they flourish?

What if a gang member with a knife came up to John and tried to force him to rob the store they were standing in front of? Does he have stored information which he can process and compare to past scenario's to be able to formalize a plan to get out of the crisis *and* not get killed?

Probably not…

Now what if Joe found himself standing in the high school auditorium giving a speech to the graduating class as president of the National Honor Society? Does he have the stored information to process and compare to past scenario's to formalize the plan *he* needs to impress everyone with his eloquent words and impeccable taste for clothes?

Probably not… It is more likely he would get arrested and thrown in jail for walking down the street with his cocky, streetwise, behavior and rough and tough exterior.

Neither Joe or John had been prepared for what they now faced.

But what if by some miracle they survived that day and the next and the next and the next?

What if they survived long enough to utilize that "information processing" and start to flourish in their *new* environment – they could, you know. Better still, what if they were actors and the situation they found themselves in were scenes from a movie – "My Cousin Vinny" meets "The Karate Kid".

Hmmm…

Information processing relies on memory – our episodic memories. Now episodic memory has a few siblings – 1) working memory; what we need for what we are currently in the process of doing and, 2) semantic memory for learning new facts and to sustain relationships. And let's not forget - 3) motor learning, (practice, practice, practice) and lastly, 4) instrumental learning - that special memory needed in behavior modification.

We keep running into this "rewards and punishments" section, don't we? It sounds like we've come full circle.

No wonder when a person loses their memory in some capacity for whatever reason not only have they lost memories of people, places and things, but also - the ability to process new situations, to learn new facts and to sustain relationships has been damaged also.

The learning curve for them has now changed and they have to start over again – like a child.

Is that why I forgot that the big box in the kitchen chilling food was called a refrigerator the other day? Uh-oh…

Guess that's another reason for us to be kind to people and not be judgmental.

Think about that while we talk about this next item our brains are capable of called homeostasis *and* maintaining this homeostasis, both crucial functions of the brain *and* a definite "must-have" for our survival.

We are talking about our physical stability now which means keeping, within a limited range of variation, things like; our body's temperature, water content, salt-concentration in the bloodstream, blood glucose levels, blood oxygen level, etc… These are the functions always needing constant maintenance - stability.

To do this our brain regulates the internal environment of our body through a series of sensors that generates error signals when a level is off, which then evokes a response and a shift back towards the optimum value – a shift towards perfect, *perfect for us.*

In addition to all the above, we also possess motivation - our *individualized* programming which causes us to behave in ways that will ensure our survival. Things like seeking food, water, shelter and a mate. Not only that but it also processes the current state of "*how satisfied* with these goals we are". And if it determines we are not will then activate the necessary behaviors to meet our need to be *more* satisfied.

Of course, that is if we really know what will make us satisfied.

Sorry I had to throw that one in.

This one is really intriguing because you would think on the surface this would be triggered by our emotions and our feelings alone - so maybe it's not totally a "brain" thing. But *this* motivation is not exactly the same as being motivated to get straight A's on your report card because your parents said they'd buy you a new bike, (I'm showing my age here).

This motivation is more encompassing and in part, a subconscious action utilizing both hormones and that famous "information processing" to "make it happen" - even when we aren't realizing it is happening.

Is that one of those "out of our control" things we were talking about before?

Ask any woman who has had one drink too many and finds herself nine months later with a little bundle of joy. Another subject for another book - we'll talk about this one at another time.

Okay, next?

Well, it's our own built-in, reward and punishment system.

Yes, "Pavlov's dog" living, breathing and operating inside of us - a perfect example of both "the brain *and* the mind".

How so?

It's the *mind* because if we do something and we get a reward that we like we are more likely to do it again. The same is true if you don't like something - you will do your best to avoid it. That's the mind.

Ironically, it's also the *brain* because when you get the reward or punishment there is a burst of electricity – a virtual lightshow of electrical activity that happens in your brain, embedding that information in your memory.

And what have we learned about that before?

You guessed it.

Structural changes are caused in the brain which affects "information processing". This "lighting up" (hot spots,) of the brain is what is caught on PET scans and which shows the areas of the brain with the most, the least and no brain activity. Fascinating stuff - especially when studying neural conditions like Alzheimer's and OCD, don't you think?

I really got hooked on PET scans and OCD about twenty years ago during my friendship with Claire, an awesome individual and my counselor when I first moved to Statesboro, Georgia. She quickly recognized my interest in the brain and when that was coupled with my slight case of OCD - look out!

It led us into many in-depth conversations. She taught me so much but sadly she passed away about five years ago, I still miss her. We kept in contact, and she was one of the first people I shared my writings with. Claire was a very spiritual person and had a unique way of blending God and science, folding in imagery and visualization to illicit profound changes in peoples' lives.

Sounds like a recipe, doesn't it? Well, I guess it was!

Anyway, back to PET scans and OCD. Claire gave me a book to read and an entire chapter of it was dedicated to an experiment involving patients with severe cases of OCD. Individuals who couldn't leave their home because of phobias or who were compelled to repeat something over and over such as washing their hands so many times that their hands barely looked like hands, but instead - raw, gaping wounds of bleeding flesh. OCD, to this extent, has always been not only a devastating and life-controlling disorder - but extremely difficult to treat and almost impossible to cure.

When PET scans became available and doctors and scientists after years of studying them realized when changes in thinking and behavior did happen it would produce a change in the person's PET scan, they got excited. They had tangible evidence - like a "before and after" picture.

They also were able to ascertain that this was not a fleeting phenomenon but that it could produce a *permanent change* - sometimes quickly, sometimes overtime. Now they were really excited!

They began an experiment to test their theory and decided to use the most difficult group of individuals they could find. Because they believed if this experiment was successful and their theory worked on these individuals - it could work on anyone.

A group of twenty patients were chosen, all had been diagnosed with severe, debilitating OCD and had been under medication and therapy for some time. In cooperation with their current therapist, a therapist from the experiment was introduced into the relationship and it was explained that a new form of therapy was being tried and this new therapy had already produced amazing results, (*setting the brain up for a positive outcome*).

Once some trust had been built up in the relationship, the new therapist explained how the new therapy was going to work. The conversation went something like this:

"We have discovered that your situation (their obsessive, compulsive behavior would be discussed), has been brought on because your brain in not telling you the truth. It is giving you false, untrue information. For some reason the correct information is being blocked and you are basically being lied to by your brain."

"Your brain wants to tell you the truth but can't, so it is up to you to not listen to your brain when it tells you to, (wash your hands every 30 minutes, 13 hours a day – for example). It is your job to tell your brain that it is dysfunctional, that you won't listen to it and that you will do the correct thing and not give in to the obsessive thoughts and the compulsion because, "You are in control - not it."

Of course, it took time, trial and error with progress and setbacks - but in 90% of the patients moderate to significant changes occurred. Individuals who had been unable to leave their homes now were able to function with some normalcy. Many were able to form relationships and have satisfying lives. They continued to need some medication and therapy, but to a much lesser degree and they were now able with the continued "self-talk" to be a major part of their own recovery.

Think about what that meant for those people.

Then think about what this means for everyone.

We are what we believe.

Our lives become what we believe.

So, if we have the power over what we believe, then "*we can change our lives*".

We can fix what is broken and compromised and return ourselves to perfect because "we were created to heal".

Our body, our brain was created to heal itself. Maybe we should practice that "self-talk" on ourselves, have a dialog with ourselves and remind ourselves that our brain/mind has lost its' perfection in the world we now live in but now *we know how to fix it.*

Remember, we were programmed to continually try to return to our original state of perfection, so to *now* succeed we must take an active role and correct our negative thoughts, ignore our incorrect thinking and overpower our misdirected brain.

Why?

Because *we know* we have the ability to overcome anything. We can't deny it any longer - *we* have the power, we always have.

And what should we be telling ourselves?

We should be telling ourselves that, "We are in charge of us and *we choose* to be healed. We choose "*our natural state of perfection.*"

So, whose voice are you listening to?

Whose voice do you answer to?

Think about that!

"Humpty Dumpty sat on the wall. Humpty..."

Stop, you say! "What am I doing?"

I'm giving you time to think about it. So go think about it, I'll come back when you're done thinking.

"Row, row, row your boat..."

"Oh, you're ready now?"

So, what is our next brain/mind deadly duo?

It's something I'm sure we all know about since we've seen and heard commercials blurting out to us about it for years - it's the affect that "drugs" have on our brain. You know those images of someone doing an "illegal substance" then the next thing you see is a sunnyside up egg cooking on the sidewalk insinuating that the egg is your brain on drugs "fried".

Well, drugs and chemicals come in all forms, shapes and sizes – and not just the illegal ones, but the prescribed and over-the-counter ones, too. They are some powerful interferers which affect both the brain and the mind.

They can have you falling down a spiral staircase which has no end or they can rescue you from a bottomless pit of darkness and despair – "one for bad, two for good".

Next...

Endorphins, I know you have heard of them before.

Well, they are a chemical – a natural chemical we have in our brains. A very important one too, as it makes us feel good, naturally. The more we have the better we feel. It's like a natural painkiller and a natural anti-depressant all rolled up in one.

Give me another jolt of that one. "Please!" "And hurry!" *"And make it quick!"*

We were created with them not only to help us feel a "sense of well-being" and to help block the minor aches, pains and minor disturbances that happen in our life but also as a *re-enforcer*.

Think about it after you exercise you feel "pumped-up", right? Like you have accomplished something grand, right? That good feeling reinforces the exercise by outweighing the work of the exercise, this way you will do it all again tomorrow and the next day and so on and so on...

But what happens if something blocks this endorphin production or stops it completely?

You guessed it.

You would feel bad, tired and achy. Basically, you would feel "crappy" and would need to seek something outside of your natural, perfect "feeling of well-being" system to feel good. You would search out and find a chemical which brings about a temporary change and make you feel "different".

But, the more you put this stuff or any stuff into your body to "feel different" the less hard your body works to do it on its own. Until one day all these artificial highs have completely shut down your endorphin-making factory. The factory has closed and all the workers have left the building *and* turned the lights off on their way out!

So, now every day you must find that chemical, that drug, that "artificial thing" or else you feel terrible. You have just become addicted. You are addicted and must have that "thing" to function.

That is what happens to a teenager who is going through that awkward stage – shy or uncomfortable with themselves and takes a drink, smokes a joint or takes a "hit" and suddenly is "the-life-of-the-party" or "mellow and cool".

They liked the way they felt - the drug was the reason they felt that way - they want to feel that way again = re-enforcement.

The trouble is that the *drug* produced the feeling which blocked the endorphins. Repeating the drug continues to block the endorphins which tells the brain not to produce anymore because they are not needed. Eventually the brain stops making the endorphins all together because it's gotten the message that they are not needed.

And technically it's true - they aren't.

The sad part is that the teenager, now probably a young adult, can't feel their real feelings with the drug. So true happiness, compassion and joy is gone – lost and forgotten, dead and buried. And in its place is an "emotional zombie" walking around, indifferent to the world around them and to the people around them able to let bad things happen, do bad things and not care who it hurts.

That's addiction.

A brain that has been fed this wrong information has sent out incorrect thinking and is just like the patients with OCD. In fact, the *obsession* with the drug and the feeling it produces along with the *compulsion* to "have to have" the drug is the definition of addiction – being OCD for drugs.

Add to it a little "denial" which the brain throws in for free to keep the addict from recognizing the very drug that used to make them "feel" - now has made them empty and hollow and is the cause of their misery.

How do I know this?

I saw it firsthand when I worked at Willingway Hospital and with our residential program, Second Chances. I have seen it too, in some of the people I love.

Ironically, once your body has learned to depend on this substance, the lack of this substance, drug or chemical in your brain can lead to serious damage, injury or even death.

Alcohol is a good example of this phenomenon. A severe alcoholic if deprived of alcohol will go into DT's – which if goes untreated, often leads to death. Let me tell you a little story.

One evening I was working at WillingWay Hospital, when one of our patients who had received treatment from us before, showed up at the door. By the time he arrived he already was in DT's – shaking uncontrollably and beginning to hallucinate.

We got him into a room, in a hospital gown then stationed a staff member with him one-on-one. I quickly called the Medical Director and he - we began the critical balance of medicating him enough to stop the DT's - but not so much as to kill him.

Luckily our Medical Director and our staff knew him well and the seriousness of his alcoholism, because at times it took more than one staff member to contain him so he would not hurt himself. Two and three staff at a time worked diligently to keep him safe from *himself* and the hallucinations he was having - terrors of bugs and spiders crawling on him, imaginary people with knives trying to kill him.

The goal was not just to stop the tremors and convulsions but to keep medicating him until he passed out so his body could rest and recover from the non-stop assault it was doing on itself.

But our friend was a special case. His DT's were so severe the usual protocols didn't work.

He was in imminent danger, so treatment went to another level - walking a serious tightrope between life and death.

Every time the Medical Director gave me an order for another injection he would say, "Call me back in 15 minutes and let me know how he is." He and I continued to do this all evening and we were still doing it when my relief came on duty. Sometime in the middle of the night after more calls to the Medical Director from the nurse on duty and more medication, his DT's finally stopped and he passed out.

Back on duty the next day had me watching him closely, as he lay semi-conscious and his frail body fought to survive. Highly trained staff monitored his every breath praying it wouldn't be his last.

He slept through my whole shift and was still sleeping the next day at 4:00 pm when I arrived. His condition - was all the staff and other patients were talking about. No one, including the Medical Director, had been in this serious of a situation before.

Our local hospital couldn't help us either as WIllingway Hospital *was* the expert on detox in the area they would call *us* with questions as to what to do with *their* patients.

Even half of the medication our patient had been given would have killed a normal person, but due to the affect the years of alcohol had done on our friend and his liver it took more than four times the usual amount just to stop him from dying from the lack of alcohol in his system.

We waited, we paced, we prayed and then while I was standing in the nurses station putting medication in a soufflé cup for another patient - he walked up to me, said he needed a cigarette and proceeded to go into the courtyard with a staff member in tow, smoke the cigarette and hold a totally lucid conversation while an astonished group of patients and staff looked on.

Amazing!

That's how incredibly - we have been created.

Created to survive and to heal simultaneously using every system, every organ down to the last cell, synapse and dendrite to do it!

Revolutionized swamp water we are not.

Perfectly and loving created we are, and because of that – we can do anything!

One last provoking thought before we leave this subject about our brain and our mind (at least for now), and it is, "Scientists believe we only use a portion of our brain."

If this is so, why is the rest of it there?

To live rent free? I doubt it.

Just as we did not know about sound waves, radio waves and electrical currents until they were discovered - I believe our brain and mind, with all its capabilities and possibilities, belong in that same category.

And the only reason we can't or aren't using all our capabilities and possibilities is because we don't know about them, yet. It's only because we are not aware of them, they are still undiscovered and hidden from us.

It's not because they don't exist.

They do exist.

Let this one circulate and percolate for a while - 'cause we *will* be coming back to it.

CHAPTER FOUR

THE HEALING HEART

You may remember we have already talked a little bit about the heart whose main purpose is to pump richly, oxygenated, blood throughout our body with its every beat. This heart is needed for our very survival and without it – we won't, survive that is.

And we've discussed, in part, how it repairs itself and creates contributories to ensure it works as efficiently as possible for as long as possible. So, we won't be talking about that again.

Instead, we are going to discover and discuss what else the heart is and what our heart means to us. And in doing this, we will be learning not only about how it heals and ultimately survives but how it can be hardened, softened, broken and, believe it or not – can signal the world as to who we are, what we think and what we believe.

It can do all that?

Sounds pretty impressive...

Can it leap tall buildings in a single bound, too?

No, it's not Superman but it does represent the part of us that houses love - that *feeling we call "love"*.

Really?

Does it capture that true essence of our soul? That soul which we can give freely to others or hold back, like "The Grinch" because we have been rejected or abandoned?

Yes, it can. It can do all that.

When our feelings are hurt or we lose someone close to us either due to death or rejection, don't we feel a twinge in our heart, the ache of pain and grief? And don't we feel a warm feeling of happiness and tenderness in our heart when we feel loved and when we love in return?

On Valentine's Day pictures of hearts are everywhere and often when we write "I love you" we add a little heart next to it, right? Is that heart just a symbol or is there more to it than that?

The bible states that out of the abundance of the heart, the fullness and overflowing of the heart; we speak words loving and kind or cutting and sharp like a "Ginsu" knife, (*paraphrased that a little*).

If that's so, then maybe it's also true that without "a heart" - a heart that can love and show love, *we* can't survive. Just the same as if we didn't have a physical heart that beats.

The separation from others, this lack of communication, the inability to be a friend or to show compassion, to give and to trust others can isolate us to the point where all that is left is a "stone-cold heart" – *lifeless and without meaning.*

And a life without meaning is no life at all - *death to the soul and spirit.*

Questions?

I know you must have some of them.

How can one person be hurt, abused, used and discarded but still seek out love and give love to anyone who needs it? But yet another person takes all the kindness and love others are willing to give but never have a kind word to say or do a single loving act for anyone else?

Is this "feeling heart" - this intangible part of us, this "invisible to the eye part" of us the very thing which is eternal and lives on long after our bodies are gone?

Maybe the answer can be found in understanding what having a heart, a "feeling heart" really means.

The Websters Dictionary defines the heart as - the core of something, the nucleus. It also gives as its synonym, the word - *spirit*.

Is this a coincidence or is it the recognition that our spirit, the Holy Spirit lives in all of us – in that central part of us, our core - *our nucleus.*

It's not something you can study under a microscope like bacteria or a virus. There are no "PET" scans for it - no autopsies or dissections of it. But it *can* be measured, observed and its' affects recorded. *And* its' aftermath is the only true test of what it has been and what it has meant for each of us – each person, all of humankind – *for you and for me.*

I had the privilege for ten years to work directly with women and men in a residential setting, helping them change their life from one of chaos and failure to one of stability and success.

First hand, I observed the effects of what the lack of or misguided love can do to a person. And what the flip side - unconditional love from God can do. It can erase mistakes, rewrite history and restore what was lost – "a perfect life on purpose".

In those ten years, hundreds of individuals walked through our doors – their lives out of control. Each and every one told their story of pain, loneliness, abuse, addictions and of all kinds of brokenness - their guilt and their shame.

And in every one of these cases, their heart – their *core* had been damaged. The person that they had been - was no longer the person they were now. They were far from perfect – far from their true creation.

But through love and compassion, structure, stability and discipline, encouragement and positive self-talk, (behavior modification) - their thinking and belief about themselves and the world around them was changed. Their confidence and self-esteem restored and strengthened and their hearts healed and ready to love again.

All this was accomplished utilizing a technique we called "inner-healings" – healing from the inside out, letting each individual heal themselves.

All human beings have issues with people throughout their lives, but in the case of our students (individuals with addictions), these issues had taken on a more sinister role - the root cause of their downward spiral of destruction.

So, for them to be able to be free from the addictive past and be launched into a future without drugs and ruin they had to be able to deal with all the pain, anger and shame, forgive and then let go and believe their life now was changed.

The process went something like this:

The first step was a conversation between the student and their mentor to identify who the student needed to do inner healings on. Caregivers, parents, grandparents, were always included along with siblings, spouses, ex-spouses and boyfriends. In addition, anyone else in their life that they had strong negative feelings for. The list could be as long as a dozen or as short as three or four. God was always a part of the list, too. And we always saved that one till last.

The student and their mentor would first pray then briefly talk about each person on the list.

Sometime during this discussion, the order in which the inner healings would be done was finalized with the easier ones always being done first, to quickly begin the process of relieving their pain and gain freedom and the confidence to build a solid foundation for the tougher ones yet to come.

Next the student would be asked to write down all the things that the person said and did to hurt them or - didn't say or didn't do that made them feel bad, hurt or angry in some way. They would work on the list for about a week and then meet with their mentor again with the goal of having the student talk about the events, feel the emotions, understand and realize how this had affected their life and lastly, confront the person.

Now the confronting was not usually done with the actual person but with a substitute. We used a large stuffed teddy bear or sometimes an empty chair if the student was more comfortable with that. Once the confrontation was over the most important part for them happened next; *choosing* to forgive that person, *choosing* to forgive *themselves* for holding on, then *choosing* to let it go and put it in the past - walking into the future *without it*.

Lastly, we would have the student destroy the list in some way - tearing it up, burying it or even burning it. Very powerful stuff - surprisingly powerful!

It is hard to imagine unless you have witnessed it with your own eyes, the remarkable effect this had on each one of our students. It was so exciting!

Because once done - the changes that happened were dramatic!

One by one the inner healings were completed rendering the student freer with each one until finally the past was fully dealt with and put to rest - leaving the present and future with a fresh page to write their story on, *not continuing to drag the past to litter up the page.*

It was all about the *choosing*, you see.

Doing this simple action put *control* back into their life - the choosing to deal with the past, feeling the emotions, forgiving others and themselves, then choosing again to let go and live in the future. This *choosing* unlocked the imprisoned heart and made it possible to heal and to live a perfectly full and healthy life.

It was no longer about shutting off the heart after the hurt or rejection just to survive, anymore. It was now about the ability to feel – to be resilient. To not dry up and die a little every day, but to face life head-on with anticipation - living, loving and healing.

Where there was once dread – now there was hope and joy. Where there once was only a shell of a person - now there was a fully alive, vibrant individual ready to reclaim their life!

That is healing – that is the "feeling heart" created for survival and created to heal.

And what keeps this heart surviving and healing?

I believe it's our purpose – our life's purpose; the reason we were created.

And the difference between those individuals who are resilient and thrive versus those who just exist?

It's our soul, our spirit; the will to find the true meaning to life, our life – our purpose; to run the race we were created for - to be the creation we were meant to be. To create the healing in ourselves - which, in turn, enables us to heal others.

What about you – why are you staying alive?

What are you living for?

Who are you dying for?

Whose life are you living?

CHAPTER FIVE

THE HEALING SOUL

Last chapter we briefly mentioned the soul and identified it as residing in our heart, more accurately in our "feeling heart".

This means there is something deeper than our heart that guides us, holds our truth – our wisdom. It draws us to our true purpose.

And that my friends, *is* our soul.

Our soul is an inner guidance system that continuously signals insight to us. And if we are listening with our heart *and* with a mind of purpose, we will be living the exact life we are supposed to be living *and* the one we were created for.

Have you ever "just known" something about someone?

Maybe it was a friend or loved one or maybe it was even a stranger, but you just knew something was wrong or *you knew* what was wrong. Or maybe you just knew a piece of information about them that you had no way of knowing.

Where do you think that came from?

How did you know?

How is it possible that you could know or would know?

But you *did* know.

The better explanation is that you *felt* it.

Your soul and their soul connected - and you knew exactly what to say or do at that exact moment which was the precise thing that person needed and it was "so good" and so profound you actually looked around to see if it came from someone else - because you knew *you* never could of thought of it yourself.

"You're not that smart".

Or maybe it was more like this: Suddenly you feel the other person's pain and anguish, their overwhelming sadness and maybe it hit you in the pit of your stomach or your heart began to hurt for them. It had nothing to do with feeling sorry for them because at this point there was no need to feel sorry for them – you didn't know yet what was wrong. So, it wasn't compassion or empathy.

You just *felt* it.

It hurt. It hurt so deep it took your breath away. You felt it down deep, deeper than you have ever felt anything before. You felt it from the deepest part of you, *your soul.*

Remember?

Remember what it felt like?

How long did it last?

Who was the person?

What did you do?

I understand this because I have had experiences like that happen to me and they were so vivid and over-powering that I knew that I knew - it was more than me. It was a part of me that was beyond what "was" me, or what I knew "as me".

The first time it happened it was over a man I loved who at that time was in the midst of a terrible drug addiction. As I saw him struggle one night, *I was overcome with a pain, so strong I couldn't breathe. It literally was suffocating me, it was pure agony.*

It started in my heart - a crushing pain as if my heart was in a vice. Then it spread to my entire body and back again to my heart. It was so overwhelming that waves of dread and hopelessness overpowered me until tears began to stream down my face. At the same time there was an inner-knowing - an inner knowledge that *this* was what it was like for *him* every day - *every single day of his life.*

Then an image appeared of two hands cradling his heart and a message, no — more like a soft command. They were my hands, and I was to love him and see him how God sees him, not how the world saw him - *or even how he saw himself.*

This image of what I was to do was acknowledgement of who I was, it enveloped me - it was *my soul touching his soul.*

This is how I believe our soul works - our soul who teaches us about ourselves and about others. The thing in us that simultaneously heals us and heals others as we physically minister to others, filled with God's power.

Another one of these experiences happened one morning when I was in church enjoying the music and singing when all of a sudden, an urging nudged, then pushed me to go up to the altar.

I tried to ignore it. I told myself I wasn't going up there because no one was up there but the preacher and he was getting ready to speak. But as *it*, "the urge", became stronger I found myself not only walking up to the altar but literally lying face down across the steps leading up to the platform.

At first nothing happened.

I remember just lying there, then seconds later I began to sob uncontrollably and then - wail as waves of pain hit me. It was more than physical pain, much more than that — it was an emotional, weary heaviness; a bone-tired, ache bombarding every muscle in my body.

I couldn't move. All I could do was cry.

I don't know how much time went by, but finally several people surrounded and supported me as I was going through this aguish. I knew what it was and so did most of the people who were there that day. I was getting ready to open the doors to a ministry where hundreds of women over the next ten years would come and live and deal with their pain of addiction.

I was feeling *that pain.*

And even more than that, I was feeling the pain of the "whosoever" out there who was shackled to *their* pain. In both these cases I was not ill, but I felt pain – I experienced it.

In reality, I was operating on another plane, in another dimension. One that I was created with, the one we all were created with. A dimension we don't yet understand and one we find hard to truly believe exists and can trust in. It is also one that we can't control.

And why don't we believe in it?

Because we can't see it, because we can't touch it and we have limited ourselves to believing only in things we can see and touch.

And there were other time, too, when I just knew something - there was no evidence of it to be true, but, yet there it was - in my head.

It happened quite often when we had the ministry, Second Chances.

You see, when you are working so closely every day with individuals with deep-seeded problems it is imperative that you have that "intangible" wisdom. Or you won't be able to help anyone. Reading about people and conditions in books will only take you so far.

These are real people with real problems, not words on a page.

It's one of those situations when you know that "*you*" is not enough. You need the other part of you, that "*you*" that is connected to the eternal stream of energy and thought that connects us all – the flow of God.

The flow of the Creator to his Creation...

It is our inheritance. It is our proof that we were made perfectly for our purpose and created with invisible things we can't see but that are just as real and just as much a part of us as our fingers and toes.

And it is in this hidden, this unseen and unknown power that will return us to perfect - our healing soul.

Again, this "part of us" cannot be found by examinations, x-rays or MRI's.

You can't read about it an anatomy or physiology book. There is no undeniable proof that it exists except for the inner wisdom and knowledge that tells us it is so.

We need to live each day allowing this soul, our soul to guide us. Did you get that?

We need to "allow" our soul to guide us because this phenomenon will not just happen to us. We must knowledge that we have it, of how important it is and that we want it to lead us. We must give surrender to it and let it overtake us so we can become all we are meant to be.

It is our connection to God – it *is* the God in us, the way He made us to be. It is our soul that keeps us "moral and ethical" when our human nature tries to overcome us.

It is our compass to keep us true - lead us to truth.

Our soul is our "heart-light" - our connection to what is inspiring, bold and provocative in us and in the world.

The soul is where we *learn trust and to trust.* The soul is where our faith lives and where our faith grows - it is where we share our faith and where faith takes us to the next level.

Our soul is where our eternal energy resides.

Our soul is our "hardwiring".

Everything about us emanates from our soul.

Our soul can't be destroyed, broken or damaged.

Our soul never dies.

Our soul exists, always.

Our soul is perfect...

CHAPTER SIX

OUR HEALING SPIRIT

Unlike our soul – our spirit can be injured, broken or damaged. It can be crushed, harnessed or caged like an animal.

Or, it can "soar like an eagle" and fly above the clouds. It can push the boundaries of possibilities and become unlimited – limitless and never-ending.

It is what we believe about ourselves – it truly is the "power within us".

What makes the difference?

Well, this is where "humanness" comes into play – ours and the people around us. In the people who have nurtured us - or not. In the ones who have either fed our spirit or starved it and the people who have either said, "Anything is possible, so go for it" or "Don't try - you will fail".

The masses: parents, relatives, siblings, teachers, coaches, friends, acquaintances and strangers - anyone and everyone you have spent time with and even the ones you have passed on the street.

All...

And this "all" have either positively or negatively affected you - and in turn, ironically, *you* have either positively or negatively affected all of them.

Remember, we are all connected - and it is that connection, even the ever-so-slight one, that makes the difference in our life.

Encouragement or criticism, inclusion or exclusion, empowerment or deprivation, a "thumbs' up" or a "thumbs down", a smile or a frown - they all mold and shape our spirit and become our spirit – become the *us we believe we are.*

It's our spirit - our character, our will, our eternal strength, our courage and fortitude. In other words, it is our guts, our grit - our determination.

The epitome of this in our society today, Mohammed Ali, died a few years ago - such a tragic loss for us. As a baby boomer I had the privilege to witness first-hand what made him so great. I witnessed him not as a re-run or a memorial - but "live". I saw him box and I saw him carry the torch, (and I don't mean just during the Olympics).

Back when there were no tweets, twitters, i-phones or facebook everyone all around the world still knew who this man was; a true testimonial to "the ultimate person standing up for what he believed" no matter the cost; relationships, career, money, family, threat of imprisonment and slander.

His unwavering spirit, right or wrong, "rose" above the racially volatile 50's, 60's and 70's and above a government gone rogue and above a disease that finally took his ability to charm us and stir us, his voice: his, *"Float like a butterfly, sting like a bee" wit* and social justice.

A true boxer, an advocate, a fighter and warrior - not just for himself but for millions…

When I listened to some of the eulogies at his broadcast funeral, I was struck with something else - something not made as public as the other things about him. This *something* that he had and this *something* that he did until he was no longer able to do it anymore - the very thing which was his true "purpose" for being here on earth: his "love"- his love of people.

This love of people that showed in his ability to connect one-on-one with a single person or a multitude and make "each" one, each person, feel like *he* was *their* personal friend - that *they* mattered to *him*.

I wondered - was it his Parkinson's from boxing, the sport that gave him the title as "Heavy-weight Champion of the World" three times, which slowed and finally silenced his indomitable spirit?

Or was it his destiny to show us that no matter what life throws at you – you can be "The Greatest" if you believe, believe in yourself and in something greater than you are?

If you believe in that *something* that connects us all - makes us "know" our importance, realize our potential and force us to move past our selfishness, envy and greed all the way to forgiveness and understanding of our "humanness".

I don't know all the answers, but I do know I am honored to have lived in a time when there were people who were willing to lose everything they had, to gain the *"everything important"* - that *everything* that truly is important.

Thank you, Ali.

Thank you for carrying the torch.

Thank you for picking up a brush and painting when the words failed you.

Thank you for your willingness to be honest, for your humility when it counted and your forethought to plan a funeral that would touch a generation that never even knew you.

Thank you for passing *us* that torch.

I guess you can see how passionate I am about spirit.

And if you're not - you need to be.

Read about Ghandi, Mother Teresa, Mandela and Biko. Get inspired and realize you are part of that spirit, their spirit – because *we are one.*

We are energy that never dies, but lives on in various forms. Energy that has existed since the beginning of time and will exist forever; that energy that has bumped up against people all along - creating change.

Because, *when you hurt one - you hurt all.*

That is the truth that most people do not understand.

It's one of those parts of us which is hidden to us – unless we search it out. Unless we find it and believe and trust in it with every breath we take. The something that, "if we don't get it" will destroy the realization of our purpose – a destruction we did to ourselves.

Something else happened about the same time which hit me profoundly – the killings in Orlando. Stupid and ignorant...

Stupid - because senseless killing no matter when or to whom is just plain stupid. But also, ignorant because it is ignorance that targets, tortures and kills people who are different.

Who says different is wrong?

Who says different needs destroyed?

Not Jesus, he loved – no matter what!

Think about it.

It's like cannibalism.

But instead of eating each other - we are killing each other which "eats" away at our society, our world and our health. This cannibalism intensifies our "imperfection" taking us further and further away from our perfection and our healing power.

If you hate others, you are not perfect - you can't heal yourself and you can't heal others.

If you hate others – you hate yourself.

If you hate others, you are allowing termites, flies and maggots to eat at your rotting flesh until the imperfection and the ugliness of your heart and soul are exposed.

We were not made to hate.

There is no hate in perfection – only in imperfection. And we were made perfect not imperfect. Our body, heart, soul and spirit cannot heal if there is hate. And because of that we have lost the power to heal others.

Imperfect - we have no power at all. We have given it away and now we are powerless – the hate has the power.

It has "the power" over us, and all we can do is exist in an imperfect, temporary body until it perishes. Our spirit is deadened, and hate is in charge. Nothing good can come out of hate, only more hate and destruction - nothing can be built.

Hate does not make a difference, only love – perfect love makes a difference, heals and satisfies our human need to be loved, included and valuable.

See the difference – understand the difference - Ali vs Orlando.

What am I saying?

I am saying that the desire, spirit and will of what one *can* do - *is* that inner power. Our inner power, your inner power – that which is one with God. And when you line up perfectly with your Creator for the purpose you were created for nothing can stop you.

It is impossible for you to fail.

That supernatural inspiration, that divine force which is infinite in nature makes all things possible. It empowers you to know that *nothing* is *impossible*.

And because, "*You can do the impossible" - you can do something that has never been done before!*

It is our responsibility as a child of God to use the spirit that God breathed into us, the spirit He gave life to – to make a difference every minute of every day.

When we feed our spirit and daily make the most of every opportunity and every challenge in our own life – that is *us healing ourselves.*

When we encourage others, lend a helping hand, acknowledge another's burden and intentionally help lighten that burden – *we are healing others.*

This healing power is within us, always. We are born with it, and it continues to exist after our flesh dies – this powerful spirit lives on. We can't see it, but we know it's there, we can feel it and others can feel it too, because it can be felt.

It is alive and able to make changes happen, make miracles happen - *to inspire.*

But we must realize this undaunted spirit requires commitment. It requires the spirit of a champion, of a lion. You must have the commitment within you to defy the odds, to never stop and never stop trying. To pick yourself up after you fall or fail and keep going - keep going no matter what and no matter how long.

Remember, it's better to break a man's leg than to break his spirit. A bone is easily mended but a broken spirit is delicate – delicate until it is strong. Delicate until it can run on its own power - until it can run a marathon. In other word - our resiliency.

Resiliency…

There have been many studies and much research done on people's resiliency, or lack of. I know, my daughter's a Psychology professor and has done research projects and she studies statistics and outcomes to try to find the reason why some people can overcome, and why others can't. Why some can rise up, and others stay down.

What are the reasons?

There's many of them: support, lack of support, resources, lack of resources, education, lack of education, positive self-image, negative self-image, money, lack of money, and the list goes on and on. It could fill a book. It *has* filled many books.

But there is really only one answer – spirit.

We all have one, and in the beginning, it was perfect because we were made perfect.

And as we have recently learned perfection is now "living in imperfection" - in an imperfect world. It's not as perfectly connected to its source as it was in the beginning because we have lost the ability to recognize and fully understand - who and what we truly are, the power we truly possess and how to use that power.

So how can we use our spirit to heal ourselves and others?

We must believe - we must believe we can.

We must believe all things are possible because the bible says so. (*Matthew:* Chapter 19)

Peter walked on water because he kept his eyes on Jesus and believed. And when he took his eyes off Jesus and stopped believing that anything was possible - he sunk, as do we.

We sink like a bowling ball dropped out of a boat. We sink to the bottom - that dark, bottomless place.

The key is to *believe.*

The disciples saw the miracles, believed and performed miracles themselves.

Our challenge is much greater since we didn't personally see Jesus do miracles, and because we didn't personally see the disciples do the miracles – so we don't realize *we* can do them.

We don't believe we have the power to do them.

But that's where we are wrong – again our imperfection is showing. This time it is our imperfect belief system we are talking about. A loose screw has found its' way into our machinery, and we have gone haywire. And the only way we can correct and rebuild ourselves so we can run perfectly again is to believe - not just a little bit, but we must believe it *all.*

It's time to take your power back!

We operate daily in our own belief system. And as such, we only will go as far as this belief about ourselves and the belief about others will take us.

We "have to" change our belief system.

We "have to" throw out the old paradigm, the standard on which we have believed and start over – start again with a clean slate in front of us.

We must trust - trust that we have the power to make miracles happen. Then, we "have to" have unwavering faith. Have the faith that "it is done" even if we don't see the results yet.

Believe...Trust...Faith

How far are *you* willing to allow your spirit to take you?

Did you ever think about why you have an imagination – why all humans have an imagination?

You don't see dogs or cats or horses inventing things, do you? Animals are trained.

Humans imagine, visualize and invent.

What if our imagination isn't just us daydreaming.

What if our imagination is the lock and belief is the key - our belief in all things possible.

And that the possibilities *are* reality - that all possibilities are our reality. And, if we live with this being our reality, then healing ourselves and healing others is normal *and the way back to our perfection.*

What if imagination *must* be present before reality can be present?

What if our imagination must *think* our reality before it becomes our reality – before it *can* become our reality?

And what if - after we think it we must believe and *feel* it?

What if it's our strong emotions – our feelings that something is real that makes it real? That we *must* experience and live from the place that *it is* real and then it becomes so – real and our *new* reality. That is what Dr. Wayne Dyer believed. It's what he wrote about in his book, "Wishes Fulfilled".

So now, how do we find our way back to oneness with God and the universe?

I believe it is the ultimate use of our body, heart, mind, soul and spirit with the belief in the infinite and the limitless - belief in this boundless perfection we were created into.

It is time to go through the portal, the doorway, and get a true glimpse of the possibilities and give yourself permission to receive.

And believe....

CHAPTER SEVEN

THE "REPLACEABLE & IRREPLACEABLE YOU"

Let's do some reviewing.

We have briefly discussed our 1-100% notion that we all fall somewhere between 1% and 100% healthy for the current time we are living in. This is reality – it's tangible.

Now the belief is when we were first created our bodies were hard-wired for perfect health and well-being for _that_ precise moment in time and place in which we were created, and for the exact purpose we were created for.

Over time our environment and the changing world around us has created a "great divide" between our natural health and well-being and what each of us is experiencing _now_. And instead of an effortless life we are forced to "work" at being healthy, finding peace of mind and having a feeling of "well-being".

Each of us "work" at this differently, and with varying results.

The ones with the least information, the procrastinators and the stubborn - gravitate towards high levels of stress, unhealthy lifestyles, unhealthy relationships and sick bodies. Not only do these people routinely keep their bodies out of alignment with their natural ability to heal - these people also keep their "loved ones, their circle of influence" sick, too.

If you have ever lived with, loved or been an alcoholic or drug addict, a person with an eating disorder or sex addiction, a workaholic or a compulsive gambler, (which is about 50% of us) - you know exactly what I mean.

This group is looking for an "outside" fix to their problem - or at least what they think their problem is.

Instead of looking inward they turn outward to substances or any new fad that promises to make them happy and when this doesn't work - they continue down that rickety, spiral staircase. When, in all actualization, they have just aided and abetted their body to be even *further* away from its natural abilities to heal - to be perfect.

What else have we learned?

Well, we've learned that another roadblock to our perfection is the constant change of the environment and the world, the global community.

Even if we get it figured out for today, who knows what tomorrow will bring? An earthquake in China, an oil spill in the gulf, out of control forest fires – these can not only change the landscape but change the delicate balance of animal and plant life that we, humans, are vitally dependent on.

Contaminated water which infects the fish that we consume, insects vital to the chain of life which first are an endangered species and then soon become extinct. Chemicals that not only spoil the environment but change our body chemistry - *and suddenly*, we aren't metabolizing foods or medications anymore. As a result, our bodies are suffering and becoming more and more ill.

How do we combat all of that?

Hold on to that last thought and deposit it in your brain somewhere safe where you can retrieve it easily when we are ready to answer that question.

That's right, I'm putting you off here for a minute because first we need to absorb a little bit more information.

You must consciously allow yourself to receive this new information, open your heart and your mind to your inner knowing - your inner knowledge. To that part of you, that part all of us we were born with which is special and unique and is the connector to our purpose and to our Creator.

That inner wisdom if we listen to it, not only keeps us in our natural state of health and well-being but keeps us focused on our path in fulfilling our ultimate purpose - ensuring we create an amazing journey along the way.

You notice I said our natural state of health and well-being and fulfilling our purpose – *not someone else's.*

Ah-hah!

So then, the pitfall to look out for and avoid must be your time spent looking at others - thinking you (we), must be like them – or *them like us.*

It's not our job to look at others and what they are doing, eating, exercising, thinking and living for. It is our job to focus on *ourselves -* to pay attention to ourselves and learn what *we* are supposed to be doing and then do it so our body is physically, mentally, emotionally, socially and spiritually ready for the purpose we were given.

This is what culminates into the "replaceable" and the "irreplaceable" you.

If you have been paying attention you have discovered already that there are two "polar opposites" working together in this book and in your life - the very tangible and the very intangible.

Why?

Because that's how we were created - we are both. And it is for this precise reason why we, (you and I) are replaceable and irreplaceable.

That is the truth of us – the secret of us, the success of us, the humanness of us; *our perfection, our god-created quality.*

What we believe affects who we are, how we live, act and react, our health and our happiness.

Our thinking, (our mind) is like a magnet. What we believe, what we think and think about the most comes to us, it sticks to us – increases. So, there is more of it - more us, the "us" we believe we are and less of the "other" us, (what we don't believe we are).

This belief about ourselves will either: keep us well and perfect for whatever comes along, or it will make us and keep us sick, so whatever comes long will conquer us - because we have "believed" it so.

The fact is, if we believe in something even if it is wrong but we believe it hard enough – we can convince ourselves and anyone else that it is the truth. The more we project our belief and never waiver the more powerful it becomes, until the lie becomes reality - *our reality.*

We must live as if what we have imagined and believed is our reality. Live it to the fullest and really *feel* it is so. Live with complete intention. Then the good news is - we can change the future - our future, and *you* can change *your* future.

We can change the present – the present which changes the future, (your present and your future) *and* the present and future for *others,* too.

That's the Law of Attraction in a nutshell and it is everything and it is *in* everything. It is the perfect example of the "we reap what we sow" principle. What we put out comes back to us and "what we believe will be".

Don't believe "too little" - too small.

Don't settle for *low* expectations because that is exactly what you will get. *You will have brought about less than you are capable of – less then you really wanted.*

I've done that before. In fact, I recently realized that I have done that all my life.

When I look back, I see myself ordering the least expensive item on the menu, afraid to spend a few extra pennies rather than ordering what I really wanted. Bought clothes I didn't want because they were cheap and denied myself of so many things and experiences all the while believing it was the wise thing to do – the "noble" thing to do. When in fact it was the exact opposite of what I should have been doing because I was just making myself unhappy, feeling cheated and bringing about more of the same – over and over.

The truth is - *I'm the one who created that present and that future which was less than satisfying.*

Me, I'm the one.

I have to take responsibility for that, and if and when I do - I then have the power to change my present and my future.

And since I've learned this lesson, I've made changes in many areas. I'm not 100% where I want to be – not quite yet. But I'm getting closer every day and the exciting and encouraging thing is I know it's already there for me – the physical just hasn't caught up with my reality yet.

Did you hear that?

"The physical has not *yet* caught up to my reality".

And guess what?

The same thing is true for you.

Yes, I'll say that again, *"The same is true for YOU!"*

Pretty powerful stuff, huh?

But there is another truth or more specifically there are other truths we must come to know if we are to fully live and operate in this life we have been given. And that is, if we don't grow in the understanding of who we really are and what we possess we will be living only half a life and continue to walk around not understanding why we are in the state of health we are in – which is a life *far* from perfection.

We will think that this is the way it is – the way is supposed to be, the way - is must be.

We will believe, "This is my lot in life, this is all there is". And we will think about our Creator in that way, too. Asking, "How can you (He), let this happen to me?"

Our life will be lived with a permanent "*why*" pursed on our lips and live a life full of disappointments, one after another.

You must start *now* embracing the irreplaceable you - the intangible part of you that can't be replaced because there is only one of you. Start asking your body and your mind to work *with* you, not against you - "To work with your ultimate purpose, not against it".

This intangible does not form collateral circulation, or have to regenerate, mend or shed. It is exactly the way it was created and continues as a steady stream of energy between you and your creator.

If you can just recognize this and live your life with intention, fully aware of your purpose and inspiring others – you will heal yourself and you will others. Then your *irreplaceable you* - is acknowledged. And it signals your body, (the replaceable you) and you can feel it.

You are not wondering why you are here and always disappointed. You *know* the "why" and as a result, you are blessed - and you are a blessing.

You are more than you believe, you are more than you are - *you are more than you can imagine.*

All we need to do is accept who we really are and that is the great "I AM" on earth. We are here to be like God, we are here to be an extension of God on earth – *God in action.*

And when we profess "I am" perfect or healthy or healed - we set into motion the alignment of our inner attitude with our spirituality, that's where the power is. When we understand this, then we will be able to release the power to turn our thoughts into actions. Thank you, Dr. Wayne Dyer again, for helping me see this.

That irreplaceable you, (the irreplaceable me) is a spiritual being and it is the spiritual being that is God. It's only our physical body that will eventually die that is our problem. Again, we are at odds with our self - we are limiting ourselves.

We are looking at the temporary versus looking at the eternal.

That's why we have such a hard time accepting and believing the truth about our spirituality. We think "we" are our physical body that will eventual die - but in fact, that body just houses us, (you and me).

Need an example?

Let's say you live in an apartment building and your apartment is on the third floor. Is the apartment building you? Do you say I am Apt. #306?

No, of course not!

You just live in that apartment which protects you from the outside elements and gives you the ability to cook, wash laundry, sleep, etc…

What happens if you get evicted from your apartment, decide to move or the apartment building gets torn down. Do you cease to exist?

Hello. Do you understand now?

I was fascinated by a movie I watched last night entitled, "Lucy" which took the idea of what *could* happen if someone *did* use 100% of their brain, and then the author made that idea into a "thriller". Unfortunately, the main character spent the entire movie using her increasing abilities to avoid being killed instead of using those abilities to make a positive difference.

Oh, well…

But guess what?

At 100% her physical body, (her shell) disappeared and all that was left was her energy - she *became* energy. Her physical body was gone, and she became part of the unseen, the universe.

She became what we have been talking about in this book.

With every increase in the use of her brain she was able to see, hear and do more and more amazing things. The bad news is, it also exposed the realization of what those increased abilities could do - if put in the wrong hands and used for the wrong purpose, the destruction of others.

Maybe that's why we only able to use a part of our brain, hmmm...

I guess God did know something about us human beings because when Adam and Eve ate that apple and mankind *knew* the difference between right and wrong and they were *able to choose* "wrong" - they were no longer "safe".

They were no longer safe in the Garden and so *we* were, (are) no longer safe.

We are no longer safe, no longer safe to ourselves and safe to others. Something to think about...

Our lives as they unfold are designed perfectly for our ultimate purpose. At the same time that this is happening we have a body, and a spirit designed perfectly for the survival and healing of our life, and the lives of others. Together these two independent but intertwined systems reflect God's true nature, his character and his heart for us - the mirror reflection of himself.

Replaceable – created to keep you going (like the Energizer Bunny), so you can realize and utilize your ultimate purpose.

And the "*irreplaceable*" you – that conscious stream of God-like energy to heal, inspire and connect with all the other God-like energy contributories and, "*Change the world!*"

So, what are you waiting for?

CHAPTER EIGHT

"THE GIFT AND PURPOSE OF HEALING"

Don't be denied.

Don't be denied of your purpose - that amazingly, glorious God-given purpose.

God decided thousands of years ago that His Creation; "You" would be created with a purpose and the abilities required for you to fulfill that purpose.

He gave you this gift.

And it is a gift!

And *even though* Adam and Eve messed up *their* purpose that doesn't mean you have to mess up yours. *Even though* they got themselves and all of us kicked out of the Garden and into a foreign, unfriendly world doesn't mean we can't learn to live within it.

Even though we have forgotten why we are here, what we are supposed to do and how to do it doesn't mean we can't remember, learn and accomplish.

Even though we can only use a portion of our brain (*because if we fully used it we'd probably be capable of destroying the world*), we can use more than we are using now and we can make a better and healthier life for ourselves and others.

We can do this - and we can heal. We can heal ourselves – our bodies, our minds and our hearts and then we can do the same for others.

It is just a matter of really wanting to do it. Because if we *really* wanted to do it - we would be capable of accomplishing anything, right?

Isn't that's what the bible tells us?

It says we can do all things, nothing is impossible - and we are more than conquerors with our Creator. That is as long as we believe we can.

"Let the weak say I am strong". *Matt 19:26.*

That is, "If we choose to".

That's a big "if".

Why is it so big?

Because it will take commitment and determination on our part - on your part and it will take compassion, obedience and sacrifice. It will take intention and trust and belief. It will take going against the grain and not being a part of the herding crowd passing you by.

It will take being bold and courageous and it will take being an individual and *"your own"* person.

Are you interested?

If so, and I hope so – read on.

First, "What is healing"?

And remember, whatever we, (you) decide healing is – it isn't just for you. It's for everyone, every human being on this planet, whether you like them or not or agree with them or not.

You have the ability and, the capability to do it, you know.

But just one disclaimer - you have to understand your purpose so you don't make a mistake or, at least make any more mistakes then you already have made.

Sounds like you are going to have to do some homework - you are going to have to pray and meditate with God. You are going to have to listen closely to what He puts in your heart and you are going to have to accept his answer. Then you are going to have to do what He tells you to do - *to fulfill your purpose.*

Listen and learn, remember and accomplish…

Now let's talk more about the meaning of healing – first for ourselves and then ways to heal and help others heal.

We realize that there is sickness in the human body, mind and heart – in all humans; you and everyone else and there is also sickness in the world, as a whole. And once you find and know your purpose, you will have the perfect and very necessary knowledge you need to heal and be healed.

The *easy* answer to, "What is healing" is *to be cured*. If an arm is broken – set it, let it mend and, "poof" it is healed - you are healed.

Seems simple, right?

The bone used its' pre-programmed instructions to heal itself. So, you're wondering, "How can talking about it be so important"?

Well, the answer is: because *you* are involved. You are part of the story here and depending on what you do or don't do will determine the outcome of the story.

Will there be healing?

And if there is healing, will it be a "perfect" healing? Or one with complications and flaws?

This is where you come in. This is where *you* are the author of your own story.

What if you interfere with the mending?

What if you don't give it the opportunity to heal correctly?

Guess what – you re-injure it.

You think you know best so you take the cast off. You use it, abuse it, the bone doesn't heal fully so you don't regain 100% use of that arm. Even worse yet, arthritis sets in with pain and limits the use of that arm some more. So, you use it less and less until you have put limitations on your life, your happiness and most importantly – your purpose.

All because you didn't do your part, you were stubborn and prideful or maybe just ignorant to the facts.

We can't just so around day to day and expect everything to be "okay" all by itself. We just can't: "do, say, eat, abuse, not use, ignore, limit, deprive, over-indulge or starve" and expect - perfection.

Yes, we have a wonderfully, tuned instrument that it is a miracle of healing and preservation.

Yes, we have an inherent survival system - but to fully be able to do our purpose here on earth we must take care of our physical, mental, emotional body so it isn't get damaged beyond repair before we have accomplished our mission – before we have accomplished our purpose.

Remember, *we* have the power to over-ride what our body and mind is trying to do to help us. We have the power to hurt ourselves.

We are a blessing - *or* a curse - to ourself.

Which are you – the curse or the blessing?

And, by the way don't allow anyone else to get in the way or alter what you know is your truth - your purpose, your reality. They will try you know. What are you going to do about that?

Let's try another simple example - this one is about healing someone else.

How important do you think touch is?

In the bible the lame and blind *believed* that if they could "*just touch*" the hem of Jesus' garment they would be healed.

His garment!

That was the degree of their faith, the greatness of their faith. So, I'd say that "touch" is a very powerful healer, wouldn't you?

I work and minister in a center for the elderly and I see so many people in the second half of their lives living with some type of infirmity and struggling for true quality of life.

As we know, in the year 2025, there is more dementia and Alzheimer's disease than ever before and one of the symptoms often is anxiety and fear. Trembling, crying, agitation, confusion, depression and loud verbalizations often make up a big part of their day.

Did you know that a soothing voice and soft touch can break through and relieve the pain they are experiencing?

Where nothing else has worked – *touch*, the compassionate and caring physical contact of another human being can heal those symptoms for that moment in time.

Yes, they were healed – *not cured*.

Sometimes we are healed and sometimes we are cured.

Sometimes we heal others and sometimes they are cured.

Think about the difference.

Again, it all goes back to God's ultimate purpose for us here on earth. This is what makes it difficult for us to grasp sometimes, mostly because *we think everyone should be healthy, happy, wealthy and wise.*

But the truth of the matter is if that was so it would be more like heaven, not earth. But we are here on earth now and must do our best to do the job God's asking us to do until our time is up and these flesh bodies no longer exist - and we again are just pure energy and again reunited with "our Source".

But until that time comes, we must keep our hearts and minds open.

Fear, doubt and unbelief – polluting our mind with these negatives and not dwelling on the good things like the bible says we should do, is contrary to our purpose.

It is our old truth, old stuff – not our *new* truth, the "who" we need to *be now*. So, it's our job to make the non-existent (what we want), our *now* reality.

We, (you) must make a shift because the belief that your problem is chronic or incurable leads to *no hope*. And believing our situation *can't change* <u>blocks</u> the self (us), from healing – ourself and from healing others.

We need to walk and live as if our body is already totally healed and not dwell on our limitations and what we perceive as handicaps.

If we can do this - then *it is*.

If we don't see it or feel it - it's because the physical manifestations haven't yet caught up with the mindfulness of being healed and being in "the perfect" health, for us.

We need to use our passion and creativeness to imagine our perfect health and well-being for *our purpose* and then just wait – it will appear.

It has to.

For if you believe something strong enough it exists in your mind, which is where reality begins. It's just a matter of time until the rest of you and the universe work together to make it so, (manifest it) bring it to fruition.

We must stop worrying, constantly running after every new fad "to gain perfection" which is advertised on television a marketing tool. We need to *just move* and go about our normal business everyday *confirming* the ultimate truth; "That we *are* healed, healthy and perfect".

Once you imagine it - it exists.

It exists in your subconscious mind

It's there already – you just need to get it into your "line of sight".

Did you get that?

Did you understand it? Do you *really* understand it?

You are in control.

And because you are, *you* decide if you can and will be healed - if you can and will heal others.

The ball is in your court, so to speak.

Your new truth – your new reality and your future is up to you.

It is up to you – happy or miserable, perfect or imperfect.

Our past has brought us to where we are now the same way other's pasts have brought them to where they are now, in this moment of time, either helping their Creator fulfill that purpose or getting in the way and interfering with that purpose.

What's your story?

Which one are you?

CHAPTER NINE

"...YOUR ASSIGNMENT"

I know what you are probably thinking, "Another person wanting to tell me what to do, tell me what not to do and how to run my life".

Actually, "No."

Next you will probably say, "People all my life have been doing that to me. So, finally I just closed my mind, blocked them out and did what I wanted".

How's that been working for you?

"That good, huh?"

Well, relax.

I'm not going to tell you what to do. What I am going to do is share with you" what you *can* do, if you want".

And if you don't, "Oh, well, it's your choice. Free will – remember? Here it is - believe, just believe.

Believe in the possibility that everything we have talked about in this book is true.

Believe that not only were we created in the image of our Creator a long time ago, but that we still have His power - the power *today* to heal ourselves and to heal others.

Believe that we still have the power, you still have the power - to return to perfect, our perfect - *your perfect*.

Next, "Read".

Devour everything you can get your hands on about the human body and how everything works – every system, organ, tissue and cell. Read how every action affects the next action. Read why eating fruits and vegetables is critical to our health and to our ability to heal ourselves.

And don't stop reading until you are utterly amazed as to how intricate and beautifully our Creator created us to be. Then, read about vitamins and minerals and why we need them. Read about why you should eat healthy proteins instead of that triple scoop, hot fudge sundae I know you are craving right now.

Read labels and *eat what you need* – not what you want. Or really, what your untrained mind (your lack–of–information mind), is telling you.

Did you get that one? Please read that again.

Eat what your body needs – not what your body wants, and soon what you need *is* what your body wants.

You will start to crave the "good stuff"; fruits, green leafy vegetables, yogurt, (we need probiotics now for digestion) and supplements and herbs like flaxseed and turmeric.

That's in the bible too, you know. Look is up. God will give us the desires of our hearts when our desires line up with *His*. I'm paraphrasing again.

Learn.

Learn why eating healthy, getting enough rest, moisturizing your skin, taking care of your teeth and not letting stress get the better of you, is so important.

Take.

Take smaller portions and eat them slowly – you will be satisfied and you will eat less and enjoy more. And take time to sit down and make each meal or snack, however small, *a dining experience.*

You eat first with your eyes.
What?

Yes, you do. What is appealing – what looks good will taste better to you, it's a brain thing.

So, do it!

Move.

Move, exercise, walk and push towards the goal of the perfectly fit body for you and your purpose. Kick in those natural endorphins and feel alive with energy to burn. Smile, laugh, dance, socialize and get out and meet people, meet the world!

Drink.

Drink in life every day and make it an adventure, make it a banquet!

It will never come again and once it's over, it's gone – you cannot get it back and you cannot repeat it, so appreciate it.

And speaking of drinking – drink more water, too. It flushes everything and helps every system in your body work better. *Remember there was no Mountain Dew or Coke in the bible, right?*

Quit.

Quit loading up on the bread, pasta, rice, white potatoes and gravies. Not only will that stuff clog your arteries, it will make you blow up like a balloon from the gluten and extra calories – especially if you slab a whole bunch of butter on it!

Explore.

Explore art galleries, museums, theatres and cathedrals.

Get your hands dirty in the soil, get them covered with color on canvas.

Write a story, write a poem, write a grocery list - remember you are writing your life.

So, go wherever your creativeness takes you.

Share.

Share and believe – don't get in the way of God's creation: which is *you*!

Plan.

Plan something - remember your earthly goals go hand in hand with your spiritual goals *and* your purpose goals.

Study.

Study your bible from beginning to end and let God speak to you about not only the way you should live your life but also about *who* you really are and about your purpose which he has given to you - and to *you alone*.

Connect.

Connect all the dots until you realize the truth. Realize the truth about what you are capable of and of the endless possibilities open to you. And connect with people, family, friends and complete strangers.

Look.

Look for opportunities to change and heal – yourself and others.

See.

See the possibilities not the disabilities. See what you *can do* – not what you *can't do*.

Search.

Search your heart, your mind and your soul. Allow God to speak to you and *when he does* speak to you, *pay attention!*

Find.

Find what you *do* have – not what you *don't* have.

And be grateful!

Mediate.

Spend time with your Creator because that's why our ancestors Adam and Eve were originally created, to commune with God.

Well, "Hello", God doesn't change and either does his principles. His desire for a two-way relationship with us, with you – has not changed. He still wants it.

Did you really think there was another reason?

Look how much time we spend on our relationships with other people. Just think what could and would happen it you spent that much time on your relationship with God. It would change your life and incredible things would happen.

Open.

Open your heart to others. See them as God sees them, as one of his children - not as you see them, flawed with all their shortcomings.

Open your mind to God - let him guide you and discover your true purpose and how you can daily walk in it.

Listen and hear.

Listen to what is being said to you and *hear* what people are telling you - what that small, still voice inside you is saying to you and then...

Do – go. And go and do.

Do what it's telling you to do and go where it's telling you to go.

It may be down the street, across the world or next door to help your neighbor. You don't have to go across the globe to do ministry – ministering starts at home *and* right next door.

Desire.

Desire what God desires and He will give it to you. He will give you the desires of your heart.

It's in the bible – read it.

This bears repeating.

And pay attention. Make *His* will *your* will.

Love.

Love everybody. That's in the bible, too.

All you need is love, (The Beatles, remember?)

Love yourself and when you do you will have a heart that can love others. Maybe you don't like what they say or do – but you can't judge them, right?

So, don't. You don't have to take part in what they are saying or doing. Be strong, and don't become part of the problem - be the solution.

Make.

Make use of that love. Love someone who is unlovable - now, that is obedience!

Love is all you need. Make every day count!

Join.

Join the human race. Go out into the highways and byways and put yourself in the position to be used by God.

Be an encouragement - encourage and empower someone else.

Heal a broken heart or heal a body part and in the process – you will heal yourself.

Put.

Put others first.

Smile first. Apologize first. Give first. Love first.

If you do this, you will be blessed. Your life will be so full of blessings you'll think you are already in heaven.

If you do these things, you will be happier – seeing everything through different eyes. You will feel younger. And you'll look it too!

You'll like yourself and others more. And you'll be able to fit in those "skinny jeans" that have been hanging in your closet for - how many years?

Exercise.

Exercise self-compassion.

Wait!

What's self-compassion? I can't exercise it if I don't know what it is.

Well, it's being kind to you self – yes, to *you*.

It's putting yourself in the same category with all the other people you have compassion for. Not harshly judging or beating yourself down, not criticizing yourself for your mistakes and frailties and *not* ignoring *your* pain.

I know you must be a giver, an empathizer, maybe even a sympathizer – or else you wouldn't be reading this book.

You feel warmth, caring and the desire to help others – why not yourself?

Self-compassion is saying, "It's really difficult for me right now so how can I care for *myself* today?"

Wait for the answer and then – DO IT!

Honor and accept your "humanness". Be gentle with yourself.

It's not an excuse or a copout. It's balancing out negative emotions and intentionally acknowledging the need to do better.

It's allowing, *you,* to put that mistake or failure in the past where it belongs, respect yourself and then have the courage to hold your head high and start again.

Open your heart to the reality that you will have frustrations and losses, it is part of life. So don't fight against it, stop struggling – *release it!*

I love this word self-compassion. I learned of it over lunch with my daughter, she is writing a paper on it along with a colleague of hers.

It's like the first part of encouragement, the prefix to encouraging yourself. It's the understanding that comes *before* the encouragement.

We all need to be able to practice self-compassion and self-encouragement. Love is more powerful than hate or fear.

And I'm not just talking about loving others – but loving *ourselves.*

Reframe.

Reframe your negative inner dialogue and help your body heal itself. Help move yourself towards the goal of "returning to perfect" for you – for your purpose.

And, be brave. It is brave to be alive and walk daily on this planet.

It's brave to search for the truth.

So, be brave!

There are two roads to take in life - one road leads to the light, the other to the dark.

As humans in the world we live in today - we will struggle bouncing between the two.

Wrestling with our self while still trying to stay on the lighted path. If we internalize the negative things that happen to us or the ones we believe we created ourselves – not only will we walk around down-trodden but we will walk around ashamed. When this happens again and again, over time we create something – *a pattern of shame.*

This pattern of shame turns into a *life of shame* which we wear like a heavy, winter coat weighing us down and making it impossible for us to see the *perfection* in us and ultimately, we are lost to the ability - to heal our self.

Self-compassion is the tool, the trait that if we possess it can break the chain of shame in our lives. It can pluck it right out and neutralize that internal battering of negativity and shame and put us back on that lighted path fully able to see the *truth*, which is "the good" in us *and in others.*

The question is: "How can I get some self-compassion?"

Or if I'm fortunate enough to already have some - how can I get some more?

Like any of the things we have talked about in this chapter, it's going to take some work over some time. Remember, God created our world in seven days – not one. So, understand it is a process, but it is a process worth your time and your effort.

You must take prisoner all negative thoughts that pop into your head about yourself – even the little ones: "Boy, was that stupid!" "I'm an idiot" "That was dumb of me" "I wish I was as smart as so-n-so" "I can't do it" "I'll never be good enough" "I don't deserve it" "I am sick" "I am too old" - and the list goes on and on.

Then take the next step.

Stop that thinking in mid-sentence and replace it with a kind, gentle and encouraging thoughts about yourself: "I am smart" "I am acceptable" "I am made in the image of my Creator and *he is perfect for his purpose and so am I*" "I can do it" "I will make it" "I am well" "I am healed".

Live in constant affirmation.

Remember, you are in the process of building a temple – your temple of self-compassion and strength. So, it's time to wear the badge of triumph!

Again, if you believe it – it will be. "If you build it - he will come" (thank you *Field of Dreams).*

We *are* what we believe. *You are* what you believe.

And we will create the world we believe we deserve.

You will create the life you believe you deserve.

Let's repeat that.

You will create the world you believe you deserve - so accept that *you "deserve"* the perfect one for your purpose.

You can have it – if you want it.

It's all up to *you.*

Know.

Know you are loved - loved by the Creator who made you for a very important purpose.

"*You*", not *someone else.*

Turn around.

Turn your life around – it is not too late. No matter how old you are or what shape your life is in now you still have time.

And whether you choose or not – you *still* have made a choice.

Remember it's not the decision we live with – it's the *results of our decisions that we have to live with.*

So, take Charge!

Stand.

Take a stand, every day. Take a stand and make it count. Stand up for what is right and practice that every day.

Understand.

Understand that life is eternal. Your spirit, which is energy – never dies. You are endless, so there are endless opportunities for you.

Visualize.

Visualize the life you want, the world you want. And do it. Do it now!

Create.

Create that life you want, that world you want.

If you believe you can – you can. You must!

Don't go to bed angry.

I have heard that one so many times and I'm sure you have too. But I never really understood the full implication of what it meant until recently. It means; whatever is on our mind when we fall asleep, whatever we are thinking about at that precise moment we drift off to slumberland, we will program ourselves to turn those thoughts into reality through our subconscious mind.

Really think about that one.

You know you just don't fall asleep and then there is nothing – just a blank spot for "x-amount" of hours, until you wake up.

That's not the way it is - your body and mind don't shut off – it keeps on running. This is the time it replenishes itself, amps up again for the next 24 hours and part of that "amp"ing up is taking what is *uppermost in your thoughts and manifesting that into existence.*

Haven't you gone to bed thinking of the negative thing that happened that day or about the fight with your spouse, boss or friend? What happened when you woke up the next morning?

It was still on your mind, right?

Do you know why?

Yup – your subconscious spent the night churning and turning those thoughts into reality – your reality. And the next time you see that person – bingo! The argument or that negative thing hits you again and it goes on and on instead of being done and gone.

So, go to bed thinking "happy thoughts", rewrite the day and make it good - give your brain something good to dwell on while your body restores itself.

And, remember.

Remember what you have forgotten. What has been forgotten for thousands of years, what our ancestors didn't remember to tell us.

Remember you *can* do all things through Christ who strengthens you.

You *can* do what seems impossible.

Why?

Because the truth is: *"ALL things are possible with God"*. "We are more than conquerors" "All things work for the good for those who love God and are called according to his purpose, (your purpose)" and "I can do all things through God who strengthens me".

I believe we were born with all the gifts our Creator has. We were born with the capability and the ability to do all the things our Creator does. *We are God in action.*

Did we lose some with the fall of man – probably, but did we lose them all?

No.

So, it's our job to discover what we didn't lose. What gifts we still have – and use them fully.

How do we discover them?

By asking God to empower us through His Holy Spirit that dwells within us to reveal what we are capable of – of every gift we possess *and* what to do with it.

Read I Corinthians Chapter 12 and read the Book of Romans.

Just think what a life *you* could create. What a beautiful tapestry it could be.

Then think, what a world *we* could create.

Imagine...

CHAPTER TEN

"ON A MORE PERSONAL NOTE..."

"Just when I thought I was out – they pull me back in."

These are Michael Corleone's (Al Pacino's), immortal words from one of the all-time great movies "The Godfather" - and one of my personal favorites. And just like Tom Hanks' character points out in the movie "You've Got Mail" – *"The Godfather has the answer for every situation in life":*

When you don't know what to do: "Leave the gun, bring the canola's".

Or, when you don't know where to go: "Time to go to the mattresses".

And just maybe the best answer of all, the "I Chi" of all "I Chi's" - *"It's not personal Sonny, it's strictly business".*

Well Sonny for the record - just when I thought I was finished with this book and getting ready to gear up for the next project, all of the above happened to me *and it got <u>very personal</u>*.

I got pulled back in. I had to go to the mattresses and now it's definitely not, a business thing but a very, very personal thing.

I'm still trying to figure out the "Leave the gun, bring the canola's" part and exactly where that fits in – but I'm sure God will shed light on that one, too.

God is a funny God – funny "ha, ha" *and* funny *interesting.*

Where to start, hmmm…

Okay, if this is the first book of mine you have read then you may not know that all my books in some way reflect people, events and situations from my life. Of course, they are about many other things too – other people, events and situations, but I'm the one telling the story.

As I wrote this book, I did share some of my personal experiences with you which complimented the "particular idea" or principle I was writing about – so it all made sense to me as it normally does.

Well, little did I know that this was not a normal situation, or should I say, "This was not *my* norm."

I didn't know that the book wasn't done – it was not nearly done.

It wasn't just that it needed edited which books always do and gone over with a magnifying glass to look for typo's - but there was a whole section, a whole principle missing. And not only was it missing but the importance of this book, which I have always known was special – *would not* be so special without *it.*

The much-needed stark reality, the "slap in the face" part, the part that is most meaningful hadn't been written yet. It would have been like a clue had been left out of a murder mystery and because of that, it would be impossible for anyone to solve the murder.

I had to write it - and it had to be about me. No one else involved – just me, *alone.*

But I didn't know that yet.

So, I edited and looked through the magnifying glass several times and I did something I had not done before, I started looking for a literary agent. I did this because I decided I was not going to self-publish this one – it was too important!

It was going to be just like one of those other books - the books I've read during my life that changed me. That made such a profound difference in my life that I made changes which impacted my life and "my world" forever.

This was going to be one of those.

I was going to help God help others.

Ha, Ha, Ha… The joke was on me because - God doesn't need my help.

I mean he uses me, (just like he uses others) to make sure what he wants done gets done – but ultimately, *he does not need my help.*

So, on September 8, 2017 to be exact, God spilled the beans. Technically it's been a few years now.

Yes, he let the cat out of bag – he had a slip of the tongue.

Basically, it was screaming and bouncing off the walls inside my head - not only was the book not done but the reason it was not, *was me. I was the reason.*

Didn't I know that the real important books did not just have good or even great information in them, but they had the missing clue – the "*It is personal Sonny, it's not business*" moment?

Didn't I know that?

Didn't I know why those books had impacted me so much?

And yes, this book could be one of those, too – but only if it was truly finished the way *God intended* it to be finished, just as he had created us in the beginning to be – *perfect.*

Didn't I know that God wasn't going to waste all this time talking to me making sure I was typing up his manuscript precisely as he wanted it typed up?

Didn't I know that? Apparently not, but I do now.

Because, once the screaming stopped in my head and the realization set in that not only didn't I know how this chapter was going to end, but I didn't know how the next chapter of my life was going to end – I got quiet. I got very quiet - and sad, very sad. So sad that I went out and bought a bottle of St. John's Wort to see if it would lift my mood.

Still don't know the outcome of that one yet – I just started it yesterday.

So, here's what I learned.

For this next part we have to go back in time about a year ago; I had already been a nurse for many years, moved more than a dozen times, raised a child and moved numerous heavy things in my life all to the point, (don't get grossed out here) but *my inside was falling outside.*

Precisely speaking, I had a prolapsed uterus and for those of you who have not had one - it's when your uterus starts to come out due to weak muscles and strain. And along for the ride come "bladder issues" – urine dribbling or leakage with coughing or sneezing.

At first it was just there, at the edge and not really bothering anybody – just sitting, waiting. But then the effects of gravity took over and showed up with its friends; discomfort, trickling, physical irritation and the constant work to stop accidents and eliminate odors. I know this all sounds very unattractive, *and it was.* It also put a strain on my self-image and my marriage and so I did what most people do, *I ignored it* - or tried to.

I did that all the while it was making its' slow descent. I did that all the while as I went for my six-month check-up with my primary physician for a mammogram and a pap-smear, (routine for us, women). I did it as long as I could until I reached my limit and decided my stubbornness had to go – it had finally lost the battle and surrendered.

I made an appointment with an OB-GYN in the hope something besides surgery could be done. Wishful thinking, because this "pessary" idea didn't work either and it was just as disgusting as what was already happening to me. If you don't know what a pessary is you'll have to look that one up for yourself, sorry.

The bad news was that the only other solution was surgery and for the sake of insurance and my checkbook I now found myself looking for another OB-GYN "in network". After much research, I finally made my choice and an appointment.

When the day arrived, I apprehensively drove to my appointment, endured *another* gynecological exam and waited for the surgery answer which I knew was coming. But what I didn't know was that it wasn't going to be just a little "tacking up", a little "lift" of the things that had fallen - but a full-blown hysterectomy, major surgery!

Now it wasn't that I wanted to hold on to my reproductive organs – menopause had been a "gift" to me but, the thoughts of surgery and recovery and general anesthesia upset me dramatically. The "being a nurse for many years in all types of settings taking care of all types of people" was now taking over. Now, *I was going to be one of them*.

This might be a good time to hit the "pause" button and add something pertinent and important. Back when everything was really 'dropping down and falling out" I decided to lose (*again),* the "30+" pounds that I have gained and lost every other year since my mid 20's.

Yes, I am one of *those*. I've tried every diet known to man and some of the unknown ones, too.

They don't work.

I mean they do work – temporarily until you, (I) can't deny the cravings any longer and you, (I) give in an inch at a time until too many inches have been added and clothes don't fit, again.

But "no worries" you, (I) have a closet full of clothes in various shapes and sizes from size 6 to size 16 for any size and season – so take your pick.

But the good news for me, and this book - something different was about to happen, something life-changing and her name was Cindy. Cindy happened to me.

Several years ago, I met Cindy, someone raised from the womb to eat healthy and to supplement correctly. Someone now in her late 50's who takes no prescription medications and has no real medical ailments - a friend, who was about to change my life and cause me to remember what I had forgotten that, "*I was created perfect* and *I was created to heal - myself*".

What did this mean? It meant that I wasn't going to go on a diet.

I didn't need to go on a diet because I didn't need to lose weight. What I needed was to allow my body to return itself back to my "perfect" weight and well-being and live a new lifestyle - a nutritional, healthy lifestyle that would last.

So, when my OB guy who was soon to be my surgeon told me the bad news, I was not only ten pounds closer to my "perfect weight" but I had more energy, my mind was clearer, (good thing) and I was feeling more resilient.

And believe me – you can't put a price on resilience. "It's priceless!"

They need to do a TV advertisement on that one and the surgery was my incentive to not just start this new healthy lifestyle - but to stay on it. Incentives are very helpful for keeping us motivated - and is an essential component in the early months of adopting a true change, a change that will last.

This is where my friend, Cindy, was again instrumental. With her help we added some steps to my plan, (Appendix 1 is the finished product) to get me ready for my surgery which was scheduled in two months.

Why did I wait so long to have the surgery?

Well, part of the reason was I needed to have enough paid time-off from work and the other part of the reason was we were expecting our yearly visit from "the state" and I needed to be there at work to help.

Now I can't tell you this was a bad decision or a good decision – it was *my decision*, and somehow all things worked out. But if I had gone ahead and had my surgery right away, I might be writing a different story - enough said.

For the next two months I exercised, prepared and enjoyed healthy foods that my "once-dulled-by-sugar" taste buds could finally taste, *and* I did all the positive things I always tell other people to do, (☺ that's me smiling).

I listened to my Law of Attraction, "The Secret" and Dr. Wayne Dyer audio tapes every day on the drive to and from work, meditated, got my head in a good place and visualized myself coming through the surgery perfectly. And to everyone that asked about my surgery I said, "No big deal" and I really meant it. This was just a tiny blip, a tiny ripple in my life - it was nothing.

I did all this because as a nurse I knew it was imperative for my body, inside and out, to be the healthiest and at its most harmonious possible. No joke. Otherwise, it would be more difficult for me to heal and "heal perfectly" which was my ultimate goal. And happily, by the day of surgery I was closer to that perfection.

The day of surgery finally arrived, and I was ready. I won't bore you with all the details, but everything did go perfectly and when I woke up in the recovery room the only discomfort I had - was from the catheter draining my "clear amber urine" as us nurses say. It's a necessity during surgery but a royal pain afterwards, my hats off to those who need to have one permanently.

A little bit of pain medication, wonderful staff and then 23 hours later (without the catheter), home I went. The plan was for me to be off work three weeks and then back on light duty – a forced vacation of sorts. I had it all planned.

My plan was to lounge in my front yard everyday visualizing I was at the beach - my "most favorite" place in the world. With magazines to read, juice coolers to drink and a smile on my face - I felt like I was in heaven. Motrin, rest and "no heavy lifting" were my best friends.

After about a week or so I was able to ride and ventured out to breakfast with a friend. After about an hour of poached eggs, sautéed spinach and sipping two glasses of water with lemon (ugh), I was a little shocked at how quickly tiredness set in. It hit me suddenly, but "no worries", just another little blip, right?

Things were going well, and I felt proud of myself – I must admit.

So, I gave myself a high-five and a pat on the back. Three weeks later found me back to work (partial days), feeling quite well except for the nagging tiredness that overwhelmed me every day about mid-afternoon.

Time flew and it was time for my monthly check up. Confidently I zipped into my OB-GYN's office so he could see how well I'd done. To be perfectly honest I probably was a little smug, I couldn't help it.

I had worked hard and my body had done what it was created to do – heal.

Remember that old saying, "pride cometh before a fall"? Well, my smugness lasted a full fifteen minutes – all the way up until I heard *the* word.

The word was…CANCER.

What?!

Where had I been?

Who said anything about cancer? Not me – not ever!

But - there it was.

The Big C - the ribbons, the months dedicated to the disease, *the diagnosis*.

Where had I been when this happened?

Well, that's complicated.

First, after surgery my doctor had discussed how everything went with my husband who was in "shell-shock" just being there listening to him, so his scrambled brain just heard biopsy and "Probably fine". The middle part flew out the window, over his head, into the crowded parking lot and down the street somewhere.

Secondly, what I naively thought was severe irritation from the protruding prolapse and a small hemorrhoid, were actually two lesions - a cancerous one and a pre-cancerous one, both in need of removal. Which now meant, yes you guessed it - *another surgery*.

How had I missed it?

How had he missed it?

How had the OB-GYN before him have missed it?

I don't have the answers – at least not yet. Maybe it was a case of what you are not looking for you don't see or "I once was blind and now I see". Maybe it is as simple as there was no need to look under what the prolapse was hiding. I don't know, the answer has not been revealed yet.

But hah! It is *interestingly* funny that just when I was about finished with this book and had begun the editing, "here comes cancer".

Of course, what you and I both know is that the book wasn't finished, there was more to say and more to understand - and, of course, more for me to share.

Okay, back to the day I sat shell-shocked and listened to a diagnosis I never wanted to hear be said about *me*.

The doc gave me the name of the surgeon he recommended for my next surgery, one he said would clearly do a "cosmetically", great job and then - promptly set the appointment. I put on my clothes, walked out the door, got into my car and drove home.

I guess I drove home because suddenly I found myself at home staring out the window of my car which was parked in my driveway.

I'm not sure how long I sat there. Minutes kept ticking by, I couldn't get out of the car - my legs wouldn't work - and either would my brain. I just sat there – my head swimming or drowning, take your pick.

My life had just been side-swiped.

I finally discarded the car for the living room couch and sat there waiting for something to happen. I don't know what I was expecting exactly - maybe the panic to end or someone to pop out of the next room and say it was all a joke.

Maybe, "Surprise, you're on Candid Camera".

I really don't know what I was thinking or if I was really thinking at all or just staring into a very deep, dark abyss. I didn't tell my husband anything that night and I didn't call my daughter, either. I guess I thought if I didn't acknowledge it to anyone else it was still my secret and not "totally real" yet and I wouldn't have to deal with it.

Denial…

Well, at least I was having a normal reaction. Great!

The next day I confided in a friend at work, a co-worker and nurse.

We'd had great conversations about God and spirituality, and she was someone I felt comfortable enough to "say it for the first time" to.

And she *was* great – supportive and positive, just what I needed. The next time I knew would be harder – my husband and my daughter - my friend had just been… practice.

I waited a week and told my husband - he took it hard like I knew he would. Even though he has been through illnesses and operations himself - when it comes to someone else, someone close to him - he has a very difficult time. He also had difficulty really understanding what all was involved – *his* denial mechanism was working overtime.

About a week later I met with my daughter who lives in Johnson City, Tennessee, (I didn't want to tell her over the phone). It all went well - she's got a great head on her shoulders and handles situations extremely well. Thank God!

Physically I was doing great and continued with my positive thinking and audio tapes, vitamins, supplements and my "super healthy diet". I was feeling better and younger than I had in years. It's funny how you can feel great and have something wrong with you and on the other hand feel terrible when you really aren't ill.

That's the power and the miracle of our "perfection", the perfect creation of us.

Our body can be fighting an enemy – a foreigner and we even don't know it's happening. Because at the same time we are doing everything we can do to help it to do its job; healthy living, healthy diet and exercise, positive thinking and giving attention to our feeling of well-being and even taking the right vitamins, minerals and supplements.

Or, we decide not do those things and in fact, do everything wrong; terrible diet, no rest and sleep, no exercise, smoking, drinking or doing drugs, negative thinking and adding stress upon stress to our lives until we find ourselves feeling twenty years older - in pain, depressed and turning into a 600-pound coach potato.

In this latter case, *we* have made ourselves sick for no reason and become our own worst enemy. And if an intruder invades our body – we have made it almost impossible for our perfectly-created body to destroy it. Think about it.

The day of my appointment with my new OB-Gyn who would be doing my *second* surgery came. I was doing okay until I drove up to the building and pulled into the parking lot - the sign on the building read "The Markey Cancer Center".

Cancer.

Again, that word. And I had been working *so* hard doing so well in staying in my denial. What a slap in the face and another jolt into the reality I didn't want to face.

I went in.

The offices were nice, the people were nice – they were doing their jobs, it's a Cancer Center, right? Everyone needs to be nice because all the patients have cancer – which now also included *me*.

And my new doc – she was very nice, too. Another examination, going over medical results and then came the conversation no one likes to hear. The one the doctor doesn't want to say and the one the patient, (me) doesn't want to hear - but it comes anyway; what the procedure will be and what it could turn into. And since there were unknowns, the "what" that will have to be endured after the surgery were yet to come.

OMG! It was worse than I had allowed myself to believe.

I was now totally out of my comfort zone and with what she had just informed me, I was going to be out of my comfort zone for quite a while. Plus, there would be more to figure out depending on on what she found when she got in there - how much cancer was there and how deep the cancer went. The "how deep" was the issue and would determine how extensive and *painful* my recovery would be.

So, we talked about the "what-if's" and set the surgery date – September 14, giving me enough time to heal from the first surgery. I slowly drove myself back to work, again I felt like I was drowning or maybe "swimming in jell-o" was a better description. Everything felt like it was in slow motion - but not slow enough to stop.

I told my co-workers and my boss since once again I would have to arrange time off and then, the hard part – going home and having the discussion with my husband. Poor guy, now he really was like a "deer in the headlights" and didn't grasp what was about to happen and for sure didn't understand "why" there were no definite answers.

The important thing I want to share with you is that I knew I had to remain calm, keep myself from getting depressed and continue with the healthy diet and healthy lifestyle to help my body heal and also fight the assault of the enemy and get ready for the next surgery.

I knew I couldn't fight *against* my body, against my natural immune system and natural defense system. We had to work alongside each other - be partners.

We were a team now. I had to know that I "know" *until I knew* I was going to be okay, no matter what.

The day of the second surgery arrived and in the predawn hour driving in the darkness we did what most couples do in this kind of situation - we argued. I know it was just a defense mechanism for both of us so we wouldn't have to think about what was going to happen, but still it was stressful.

Again, everyone at the hospital was great, again my surgeon and her staff were great. And six hours later, found me in the recovery room - opening one eye and then the other evaluating how I felt and wondering what surgery had actually been performed.

Again, there was the catheter I hated and again the IV was painful in my hand, but the astonishing thing was this time I was totally alert and refreshed. No brain fog or slipping in and out of thought, space and time.

I felt great!

The brain, what an extraordinary machine!

Of course, the pain medication from surgery had not worn off yet and when it did I realized just how challenging the recovery process of *this* surgery was going to be. The good news was and still is, (yes, there was a bright spot as my surgeon reminded me in our post-op conversation a few hours later) the cancer had not been deep.

It was as she had thought and even though the incision was a big one, (taking out both the cancer and the pre-cancerous lesions), it was the best-case scenario that could have happened.

Thank you, God.

Now it was *all up to me* and my "created to heal" body. I am what I believe *and* what I believe will happen.

At home walking slow was okay, standing was great and even lying was tolerable, as long as I didn't move. But going to the bathroom, (I'm trying to be delicate here) was gruesome. And you, have to do that quite a bit, right? That's right, the old U & R - urinate and defecate.

I remembered back to the times I had taken care of patients with incisions in sensitive places. Boy, do I have a deeper sense of compassion for their struggles now!

Due to the removal of the two lesions and where they were located, my skin was not only pulled taunt but that big, long incision would need meticulous care. It felt like full-time job, just to do the daily care and feeding *of me*!

I must admit I was getting somewhat down-hearted.

I kept trying to see the humor in it. It wasn't funny but, I am sure I looked funny doing some of the things I had to do to take care of me and "it", (my very tender bottom). But knowing I had the power to heal myself got me through and not did it just "get me through" - it changed my life!

The day after I returned to work was my follow up appointment with my surgeon. I hadn't heard from her office which made me slightly nervous, but I tried to put that in the back of my mind very close to my "denial drawer".

In the examination room after the preliminaries were over, she handed me the pathology report and then explained why she had not called me - she wanted to wait until the weekly pathology team meeting to get some clarity before we talked.

Hold on, wait a minute – "the" news was bad?

Now what? To cut to the chase, I had to have another surgery. *Now* I was discouraged.

She was apologetic - but it wasn't her fault. Really, it wasn't.

All the indications when she did my surgery pointed to the fact that she had gotten everything but, the microscopic evidence said something quite different. It's story said that on the very edge of the incision - a tiny bit more needed to be removed to be 100% sure that all the cancer was gone. Well, of course it had to be done - we needed 100% of it to be gone.

But again, there would be the recovery period before they could schedule the next surgery and of course, there would be the recovery from that. The only glimmer of light was I would not have to stay overnight in the hospital, I could go home from the recovery room. But still, three surgeries in less than five months? Three times under the knife and three times under general anesthesia - that worried me.

I left her office dragging my feet and feeling weary. I knew I couldn't allow myself to wallow in self-pity *too* long - it doesn't help. But it was hard, intellectually I knew everything that I've shared with you in this book is true - I just needed for my heart and my emotions to catch up with it. What I needed was a day or two to wallow, so that what I did - I allowed myself to be sad, mad, frustrated, and negative for exactly two days and then I stopped.

Enough was enough and "dang it, I've had enough."

Again, explaining to my husband was difficult, the stress was getting to him, but my daughter was great and so were my co-workers and friends. Remarkably enough this next thought hit me, "God had given me an opportunity to share all of this with you." Wow!

This realization helped me "rise above" and understand more fully what I was going through and just how much we can control our existence; good or bad, recovery or not, returning to our perfect or not - healing or not.

Well, now I really was determined!

Some of you may call it stubborn, (I've been called that in the past) and others have called it something else - but the tenacious, scruffy-little-dog part of my personality kicked in and propelled me into the next surgery now scheduled for November 10th.

Again, everyone was great and again I woke up from surgery in the recovery room wide awake and alert with an intact mind. Thank you, God *again*!

But this time I was cold - I mean "really" cold. Even covered with a thermal heating blanket with warm air pumping into it - I was freezing. And "Hey, why did I have this special warm and cozy heating blanket on me anyway?

The answer to that question was - they couldn't get my temperature up.

Hello, "Had I missed something"?

It appears my core temperature had gone down, and it didn't want to come back up, bad, bad baby. Was it stubborn or lazy? Was it tired from too many surgeries?

Or maybe, just maybe the cooler body temperature helped preserve my brain?

I don't know. They really didn't know either but after about an hour enjoying my new friend, the blanket, my temp came up enough to say I was "recovered" and could go home. And I did.

Each of my surgeries was different and each had its own set of challenges and its own "uniqueness". I guess that can be explained by all the ways in which our bodies, (my body) was created to be perfect, work to remain perfect - and to heal itself.

But very importantly, I do know - that if I hadn't done everything I knew to do to get my brain, mind, body, heart, soul and spirit into the most perfect position and condition possible - *"I could never have come through this period of my life and make it through to the other side"*.

It was for my survival that I had to know all of this - and it is for *your survival* that you need to *"get this"*.

Yes, my bottom is still tender and recovering from the attack (remember that's what my body thinks happened), that I got attacked three times and its' job was to protect me, send armies to fight for me, move energy and resources to different parts of my body to sustain me and send out the radar and sonar to search and probe for new enemies for me.

And that's what it did - it did it all *for me*. Automatically, on its' own, I didn't have to tell it a thing. And along for the ride - came some wisdom, compassion and understanding - knowledge, realization and questioning.

Incredible...

And the last incredible thing, a week after my surgery my pathology report came back perfect - *cancer-free!*

"My miracle: my body returning to its' perfect, purposefully - created to heal itself."

I am a cancer survivor.

I am a survivor.

You are a survivor.

So - *"What are you going to do about it?"*

CHAPTER ELEVEN

THE HEALING ENVIRONMENT

I wonder how many of you at this point have thought, "Does she realize she has forgotten a whole other level of survival and healing?"

The answer is: yes and no, I almost did.

Remember in the beginning when we discussed how Adam and Eve were created "perfect" and, into a perfect world - and then they blew it, got thrown out of the Garden and forced to live in a hostile world?

Well let's think about this for a second. God created everything perfectly; he created the earth, oceans, aquatic life, animals, reptiles, trees and plants - all living things. And guess what? He created them perfect and then, God created us.

Keep following me here.

So, since there was no Garden of Eden for Adman and Eve - neither was there one for anything else. All those things that were created perfectly were no longer in the Garden either, but they were still perfect for the perfect world - which now didn't exist. Hello - they weren't meant to be in a hostile environment either.

God took pity on us humans and sent prophets and sent those who inspired what we call the bible to help us, help us maneuver this world so we would have the knowledge to do the right thing for ourselves and others, but have you noticed something strange about the bible?

No?

Well, here it is "Where are the instructions to take care of the animals"? Or the plants, trees, reptiles, etc., (I think you get the picture). There are only instructions on how we should treat ourselves and others - humans.

Why?

Simple - everything but humans were created "instinctual", perfect and pre-programmed - unlike us. You see instincts are beyond thought - they just are. They can't be damaged by too much sugar or lack of exercise.

And yes, we too, have programmed through our initially, perfectly created body - the difference is, we can screw it up.

Really let one sink in a while. When you do, you will realize it's not just *us* trying to return to perfect - *it's them, too.*

And then think about this one; all those things - trees, plants, birds, insects, reptiles, animals, fish and the environment were created just for us to survive *and to heal.*

Synergic, unfortunately when Adam and Eve fell from grace - so did all of they and without a playbook or instruction manual - whoops.

Conclusion?

If the environment, animals, plants, trees, flowers, etc. are damaged they can't help us, they can't heal - but they keep trying to return to that perfect, instinctually. They keep trying to mend the partnership between us - but we keep polluting it, figuratively, and actually.

If we are to work towards returning to perfect and unleash our ability to heal then we have to give ourselves a major reality check. We must realize we can't do this unless we do it in *conjunction* with the "everything else". We need to create a healed environment just as we can create our own lives and assist our bodies to return to perfect - so can we do the same with our immediate environment and the creatures in it.

We must stop living in a bubble. We must stop ignoring the truth and the signs our planet is dying.

The world is our workspace, our playground - we must heal the eco-structure that has been damaged. We must stop the extinction of insects, plants, animals - all wildlife.

We must do whatever it takes to make this happen - *protest, walk, sit, yell, shout, twitter, tweet and blog.*

We must crusade for it - otherwise we are dooming ourselves as we are still inhabiting this planet and we are also dooming the future for those who come after us.

We must respect ourselves, others and every living thing which includes the earth - dirt, sand, water and air!

You must carry this with you like a banner, like the flag of your country - *the flag of this planet, earth.*

This is important - too important!

Remember *you* create your life which includes everything around you.

Take responsibility!

You did this, too!

We are what we believe, we have what we believe we deserve.

Do you believe you deserve a healthy body, mind, soul and a healthy space to live that perfection in?

Do you?

Only you can choose.

So, what is your choice?

EPILOGUE

...ENDURANCE

Mind...body...spirit.

The ultimate "connect" which enables us to "recover" to perfect health and well-being.

Self-repair...rebalance...realignment.

The ultimate "connect" that enables us to correct the disturbances that have been hindering our ability to do our work to completion.

Intention...inspiration...visualization.

The ultimate connect that unleashes the power within to overcome what has been denying us the full access to our inner wisdom.

Believe...faith...trust.

Three out of four of the most important words ever thought of, written or spoken with the fourth being - love.

The only prison we ever truly experience is the prison our mind creates. So think freedom, think abundance – and, think of the endless possibilities.

Never stop.

Never stop wondering, learning and discovering.

But "*do stop*" and learn what you have discovered and remember to "smell the roses".

Focus your energy and unleash the power you have been ignoring because of stress, worry, unbelief and misguided negative ideas about yourself and the world. Focus on creating your environment, your world - holistically.

Stop putting up walls to protect yourself from everything you perceive as bad. Remember perception is just that - perception, *but the truth is the truth!*

What?

Those walls are now blocking out the good – they are blocking your line of sight to all the good things there are.

So now your thoughts, ideas and wishes - revolve around the negative energy in your life instead of the positive - until *you* become part of that negative energy and physically, mentally, emotionally and spiritually make yourself sick.

You have created that "sickness" and you have cut off the supply of "perfection" - your perfection *and* you have cut off the *supplier!*

You need to neutralize your obsession with those negative influences and celebrate only the good and the positive. By doing this the positive energies will continuously create healing around you; *for you and others.*

It is impossible for you to fail because you have everything available to you to create your healing and re-create your "perfect". The healing power is *always* with you – it always has been. Now is the time to wake up and wake it up!

"Wake up!" *Wake "it" up!*

You are powerful in yourself, God created you, this way when he "breathed life into you". This power is just waiting for you to acknowledge and align yourself with it and the source, *your source.*

Think of it, unlimited power to your own infinite natural universal mind. Having universal energy to unleash your ability to believe and experience total, harmonious freedom.

Let that one really - soak in. Take your time.

"And speaking of time" - don't worry about it!

Time is just an illusion, you know. You can slow it down or speed it up - your choice. It's your connection to the universal source and that is eternal; and eternally time does not exist.

Don't.

Don't do things to block your body's natural defenses and healing power. Don't block your body's longevity - *don't get in the way of your perfection!*

So now that you know you have the power to write your own story, what are you going to do about it?

His breath, his spirit - from him into us; we are part of his spirit and as such have the same power within us.

How have we used his spirit and the body given to us?

How have you?

Have we used it - in the *intent* - it was given to us?

Have you?

Oh, "by the way" did you think I forgot about the two things I told you we would discuss later?

Nope, here they are –

First, the answer to: "Us, humans only using a small to medium amount of our brain capacity."

My belief is this un-used portion of our brain is available for us to do the things we were always meant to do – but have forgotten. And what about all those teachings *not* passed down through the generations to help us know what we are capable of?

Here are two examples: healings of many different kinds, and the reading and exchange of thoughts, (mental telepathy of sorts). I do wish I knew everything we - are capable of.

If we were made in God's image, and the bible says we were, then we have not only *his* characteristics but *his abilities*, too. Think about that!

So, let's talk about the radio and TV, two things we all can relate too.

Remember they were just "*invisible waves un-used until we discovered them and started using them.*"

Well, why can't there be more?

Why not?

Do we honestly think there are only those two?

What if there are a few more?

What if there is a hundred more? Just think what that could mean, think what we might uncover. Think of what we would be able to do and experience.

Can we transport ourselves? Great question, I don't know.

But I do know there have been thousands of reports of individuals who through meditation believe they have, and thousands more who know someone who believes they have experienced transport to another space and time.

Is it a true, physically transference, an intellectual one or a spiritual one?

Again, I do not have that answer, but I believe anything is possible.

Can we move objects or create a situation to happen?

Again, the reports of these things happening range high in numbers. Twice myself I have been in a serious, gut-wrenching situation and willed and prayed with all my heart, (with everything there was in me) for a particular thing to happen. And in both those situations, within 60 seconds - it did.

I call both of them miracles - and they were.

Were they miracles from God or did "I" will it to happen? Or was it a combination of both, or something else?

Again, I don't know.

All I know is they happened - both very critical situations in my life regarding family. And the intensity and anguish with which I prayed, willed and believed was at a level I never reached before.

Could I do it again?

I don't know. Honestly, I hope I'm not in another one of those situations where I need to find that out.

Okay, next —

That oil spill in China. What are we supposed to do?

Nothing...

Unless your purpose has something to do with it and then you must listen to your spirit. It will let you know what to do. Otherwise, forget it and move on.

Don't worry about things you can't control.

Take care of the things God has put in your path for YOU to do.

Let someone else's purpose be taken care of by *that* someone. Don't interfere with *their* purpose. It's called boundaries and everyone needs to read and understand more about *them*.

Keep focused.

Focus on you and where your inner knowing is steering you — leading you, nudging you.

Why?

Because *you* are the only one who can fulfill your purpose and without "your purpose being fulfilled", the world will be less perfect than it could be.

And maybe that "rest" of our brain is there for our imagination. It's there waiting for us to turn our wants, needs and desires into reality.

So be curious, invest, create — be an entrepreneur.

Be a thinker. Ask why and then, ask "why not".

Think about it.

Know who you are, "Claim your inheritance"

P.S. I've been cancer-free for seven years!

ASK + BELIEVE = RECEIVE

THE POWER OF LIFE RECOVERY

BELIEF + FAITH + TRUST + FORGIVENESS = POWER

MY WORKSHEET

Who am I?

Why am I here?

What is my purpose?

What am I supposed to do?

Who, what where, when and how?

What do I want and how far can my imagination take me -

RECORD KEEPING

Realizations -

Healings –

Miracles –

SUGGESTED READINGS

"The Secret" by Rhonda Bryne is a book about the Law of Attraction". Read the book and get the audio tapes too, so as you are driving you can let it soak in.

Dr. Wayne Dyer – read as many of his books as you can. All of his material is great and he has the gift of not only changing your life but sparking you to *want more*. "Wishes Fulfilled" and "Intention" were two of my favorites - he has numerous books and CD's on the Law of Attraction, too!

Joyce Meyer books, tapes, videos and DVD's, - get your hands on all and any. I've seen her several times in person, and we used her materials in our ministry. She is bold, down-to-earth and will get your attention - and *keep it*.

"Boundaries" by Dr. Henry Cloud and Dr. John Townsend is a book I suggest everyone, for any reason whatsoever read. I honestly didn't know I had boundaries issues until I read this book and realized I did. This book was a life-changer for me!

"The Mom Factor" and "Always Daddy's Girl," are, must reads. Again, I didn't understand "me" until I read them both. I think you will find this to be true for yourself too.

"Search for Significance" by Robert McGee is another great one as is "The Anger Workbook". We all have anger issues, even those who don't think they do, this one will shine a spotlight on it.

And of course, - "The Bible". Read it again and again, it will show you something different each time you do. Read different versions, I read and quote the NIV, but that's me - expand your world and let God speak to you.

Why?

Because you are in a different place in life each time you read it and it will help you in different ways in any and all situations – including the new one you are in now.

That's why they call it a *"Living Bible."*

It *lives* along with you and teaches you all through your life.

Printed in the United States
by Baker & Taylor Publisher Services